Susan Wadia-Ells is a writer, teacher, consultant, and longtime activist for children's services, international affairs, and women's issues. She is the adoptive mother of a ten-year-old son, Anil, and lives in Putney, Vermont.

For Naomi who loves true stories. Wishing you a rich 16th year.
Love,
Mummy
6.2.04

THE
ADOPTION
READER

Birth Mothers, Adoptive Mothers and Adopted Daughters Tell Their Stories

SUSAN WADIA-ELLS, EDITOR

Published in Great Britain by The Women's Press Ltd, 1996
A member of the Namara Group
34 Great Sutton Street, London EC1V 0DX

First published in the United States of America by Seal Press, 1995

Acknowledgements regarding previously published material appear on page 283.

British Library Cataloguing-in-Publication Data
A catalogue record for this book is available from the British Library

ISBN 0 7043 4495 5

Printed and bound in Great Britain by BPC Paperbacks Ltd

Editor's Acknowledgements

Many people helped me during the two and a half years it has taken to compile and edit this collection. First of all I give thanks to the more than three hundred women who submitted essays and stories for consideration. I also want to express my deepest gratitude to the book's contributors for their willingness to embark on transformative journeys as they wrote, revised or edited their pieces.

I am grateful to Joan Laird and Leah Bratton who planted the original seeds for the book. In addition I extend thanks to my friend and colleague, Joline Godfrey, whose 1992 book, *Our Wildest Dreams*, made me jealous enough to finally get up enough nerve to write a book proposal, and to Larry Nevin, who shares the mothering of our child, and in doing so, helped make this book happen.

To the women of Seal Press, especially Holly Morris, my editor, who, oh so gently, and always with an uplifting spirit, led me through the book-creation process and to Cathy Johnson, the best copyeditor this side of the Pacific.

To my teachers: Rhoda Linton, Joan Laird, Mary Mason, Minnie Bruce Pratt, Laurie Alberts, Anne Bewley, Anne Black, Natalie Goldberg, Marian Ells Sharp, Nancy Bereano, Eva Mondon, Melanie Brown, Clarissa Pinkola Estés, Mary Belenky, May Sarton, Tillie Olson, Helene Shik, Anne Janeway and Marty Moscript.

To Judith Sutphen for always being there as friend, editor and colleague and to my friends and advisors: Katra Faust, Cynthia Gramer, Mary Mitchell, Kim Crawford Harvie, Marnie Crawford Samuelson, Carol Levin, Lynn Martin, Anne Glanz, Nan Heminway, Wil Hastings and Liz Wilson.

To my journal-writing group, to the many women who have written with me in my journal-writing workshops and to the members of the "Brattleboro Women's Writing Workshop." I give thanks for helping me become a writer and editor.

I thank Joanna Espy, Joy Wallens, Harriet Rogers, Feron Bratton, Debbie Tewksbury, Greg Bolosky, Nancy Braus, Judith Bush, Ann Clark, Ira Wilner, Beck Paffrath and Barbara Grier, along with the staff of Press On; the Putney Post Office crew and my friends at the Southeastern Vermont Regional Library for their ongoing good spirits and critical technical support.

For shelter, when it was needed, I thank Tim Mayo, Tamara O'Rear, Bob and Libby Mills and Beverly Alberts.

To Selma and to the past animal spirits who have cared for me all of my life.

To Anil, who has learned to live with "the book," but who is nevertheless overjoyed that "the book" is now finished.

And finally I remain forever grateful to Joan Hastings, Freda Rebelsky and to my mother, Betty Ells, for their belief in this project, for their financial support and for their profound friendship.

*This book is dedicated with love and gratitude
to my mother, Betty Ells, to my son, Anil,
and to Anil's birth mother,
a woman who, although unknown to me,
has become a source of great power in my life.*

Contents

BIRTH MOTHERS

ADOPTIVE MOTHERS

ADOPTED DAUGHTERS

Foreword to the British edition

The Adoption Reader is a welcome addition to the rather small body of literature which, by drawing on the direct experience of its contributors as birth mothers, adopters and adopted people, gives a real insight into the experience of adoption. Although the practice of taking legal and practical responsibility for the upbringing of a child born to someone else has a long and, for the most part, honourable history – examples are to be found in the early myths and legends of most cultures – modern adoption with its complex legal framework has been with us for only about 70 years (since 1926 in England and Wales and 1930 in Scotland). Until recently, the participants were encouraged to treat it as a shared secret and, by implication, something that is best not talked about – an attitude we had in common with earlier practice in the USA. The shortage of personal accounts of being adopted, or of being a birth or adoptive mother is one of the offshoots of this secrecy, and one to be regretted. While 'how to do it' books and learned texts about adoption policy and practice both have their place, nothing can quite match the contribution made by those who write of their experiences and feelings. When a new book comes along which – like *The Adoption Reader* – brings contributions that are so thoughtful and wide-ranging and in which each writer talks to us with such directness about the bad and the good aspects of their experience, anyone with an interest, personal or professional, in adoption will welcome its arrival.

Although much of the material is about the adoption experience in the USA, the similarities to British adoption are striking. While the legislative framework is, of course, different in many respects, the personal aspects – the joys and regrets, the practical and emotional concerns and even – sadly – the poor practice amongst some of the professionals – will ring bells with anyone who has been involved in adoption in the UK. What comes across clearly from these pages is how good adoption can be as a way of caring lovingly for children who aren't able to grow up within their original families, and how devastating it is when something goes wrong.

A key theme from just about every writer is the need for openness and, conversely, the terrible toll that secrecy can take. Closed records are still a problem to wrestle with in some American states and were a major issue in British adoptions too, before the law was changed in the Adoption Act 1976. Until that time, in England and Wales adopted people had no right to any information about their original families and circumstances. Although the more enlightened Scots had always allowed adopted people to acquire their original birth certificate once they reached the age of 17, in reality throughout the UK secrecy was the norm until practice began gradually to change in the late-1960s. Adopters were rarely given much information about their child's background and it was not unusual for the adoption worker to suggest that the past was best forgotten. Phrases like 'fresh start' and 'clean break' were commonly heard and adopters were often led to feel that any curiosity on their child's part about the past indicated that all was not well in the adoption. Many people who were adopted in those early days discovered their status in traumatic circumstances – when it was introduced as a reason for their misbehaviour, for example – 'you get that from your real mother', or when going through family papers on the death of adoptive parents.

For birth mothers too, the clear message was that relinquishing her child for adoption was something best kept secret and quickly forgotten. Although practice has gradually become more enlightened, it is really only in the last decade that birth parents have felt able to speak out about such unrealistic and uncaring expectations. The Adoption Act 1976, while welcomed in general by most birth parents, reinforced for them the idea that they were less important than the other participants in the adoption, by giving adopted people and adopters the rights of access to information which was denied to birth parents. Now birth parents are gaining strength and recognition from coming together to express their concerns about practice past and present, and pressing for further changes in the legal system.

In parallel with changes in the law, we were seeing improvements in adoption practice (which, indeed, inspired much of the new legislation). The impetus for improved practice came, in part, from the personal stories of those who had been through the adoption experience; those of us who work in adoption owe a big debt to individuals who – like the contributors to *The Adoption Reader* – have had the courage to share their experiences and their feelings. The other main reason for the development of new approaches was the changing profile of children needing adoption. Most obviously, in Britain as in the USA, there was a huge decrease in the number of babies whose birth parents sought adoption for them – improved contraception and greater access to abortion meant that fewer 'unplanned' babies were born, while changed social attitudes allowed more single parents to opt to bring up their child alone.

While this affected both Britain and America, the overall effect has been somewhat different – in Britain, the number of children being adopted each year has fallen to around 8000 (from a peak of nearly 30,000 in the mid-1970s) and very few are infants. More than half of British adoption orders involve children over five years of age, while less than a 1000 each year are under one. This, inevitably, means that there are many couples in Britain whose dream of adopting a baby will not come true. In America, the 'shortfall' has, to some extent, been met by turning to other, poorer countries as sources of babies for adoption. Stories such as 'Latent Tendencies' and 'The Anil Journals' in *The Adoption Reader* reflect on some of the concerns about the appropriateness of inter-country adoptions and the difficulty of weighing up the benefits to the child of a comfortable life in another country against the losses (s)he will have – of country, community and culture. Studies of inter-country adoptions make it clear that, while the child has a good chance of growing into a capable, physically healthy adult (which is no mean achievement given the condition of some children when first adopted), the experience is by no means problem free and can result in young people whose behaviour demonstrates worrying levels of insecurity and anxiety and who seem to feel 'at home' nowhere*.

The unavoidable facts that most inter-country adoptions are transracial and/or transcultural and many are 'closed', either because the child's country of origin adopts that practice or because many children have no record of their parentage and heritage, also creates difficulties. As the norm

* See, for example, Hoksbergen, *Adoption in Worldwide Perspective*, Swets & Zeitlinger, Netherlands, 1986.

becomes openness and heritage becomes something to value, the lack of information for children from overseas becomes one more reminder that they are 'different' and isolated from their origins. Combined with evidence that some children become available for inter-country adoption in very dubious ways – through kidnap and coercion, for example – has led to a very cautious approach to overseas adoption amongst British adoption workers. As a result, children being adopted from overseas form a very small minority of all adoptions in the UK – usually less than five per cent each year.

In the United States, transcultural and transracial adoptions are relatively common. As a result, because the overall number of adoptions in America is so much higher (60,000 compared with 8000 in Britain) and the proportion from overseas is three times as high at thirteen per cent, there are about as many US adoptions involving children from abroad as the total number of British adoptions. This, nonetheless, leaves the overwhelming majority of adoptions in both America and Britain which do not involve either inter-country adoption or healthy white babies. As the number of such babies decreased, the attention of adoption workers turned to the children who had previously been deemed 'unadoptable' – those who were past babyhood when their need for adoption became evident, those with disabilities and those with one or both parents from a minority ethnic group. By and large, the recognition that the first two groups were adoptable – and a lot of hard work – was enough to get them into adoptive families. It can still be difficult to find adopters for a belligerent 15-year-old boy or a five-year-old with severe multiple disabilities but the days when they were simply not considered for adoption are – or should be – long gone.

The history of adoption efforts for black children has been more complex here as in America. For the first 50 years of modern adoption in Britain, adopters were overwhelmingly middle-class and white and black babies were almost always left to grow up in the care system, if their original families could not care for them. The first wave of reaction against this practice in Britain coincided with the 'melting pot' approach to improving race relations, which reached its peak in the late-1970s. Since we were all alike 'under the skin' what could be better than for the black babies to be adopted into non-racist white families. Many black children benefited from this, in that they grew up in loving adoptive families rather than in institutions and the loss involved – of their culture, language, religion and family heritage – only began to be evident as the adopted young people moved out of the protective circle of their immediate families in adolescence. As they moved on into adulthood, increasing numbers returned to their adoption agencies not only seeking information about their original families but also trying to convey to the agency staff their feelings and experiences around being transracially adopted. By that time, a general consensus had begun to emerge in Britain that cultural differences were valid and valuable and that placing black children in white families, however well meant, might not be the best way to build a harmonious community. In Britain today, transracial and transcultural adoptions are often seen as best avoided, other than in exceptional circumstances and most effort is directed at recruiting a diverse group of adopters to meet the variety of needs children have, including those arising from their heritage.

Diversity of adopters is one area where – to judge from *The Adoption Reader*'s introduction – practice has moved further in Britain than in the USA. At present, the only legal limitations on who may adopt are age (you must be over 21) and capacity (you must not have committed offences against children) and agency assessment processes centre (at least in the best agencies) on the applicant(s)' ability to parent a child. The scales are still somewhat weighted towards married couples, in that joint applications are only legally accepted if the two prospective adopters are married to each other. However, unmarried partners in stable relationships are welcome as applicants by most agencies, particularly as adopters for children with special needs, and assessed as a couple in the usual way. Practice also tends to favour two parents over one, partly because that is very often what the birth parents wish for their child. However, those recruiting adopters operate largely from an inclusive stance – 'let's look at what you can offer a child' – rather than seeking to rule out those that do not conform to some imagined ideal. Sadly, this approach – which has enabled us to find suitably unusual parents for some very unusual children who would otherwise have grown up in care – is under threat. Proposals for new adoption law threaten to reinforce the view of married couples as the ideal to such an extent that we risk losing the diversity amongst adopters that has enabled so many 'square pegs' to be happily adopted over the last 20 years and so many different adults to experience the fulfilment of adoptive parenthood.

Legislators and others with an influence on future adoption policy and procedure should be encouraged to read and learn from the contributions in this book. Nothing could more clearly indicate the need for sensitive and informed practice, nor the benefits to be had from a flexible approach and diversity in those who take on the difficult but rewarding role of adopter.

Chris Hammond

Chris Hammond has had a personal and professional interest in adoption for more than 20 years. For much of this time she worked for the UK co-ordinating body, British Agencies for Adoption and Fostering where she was director from 1990 to 1995. She has been particularly involved in developing adoption services for children with special needs. One of her main concerns is that the legislative and procedural framework should encourage good practice in adoption, rather than obstruct it.

Introduction

Adoption, like motherhood, has always been a woman's issue. It is women who give birth, and women who have had their birth children taken from them because of cultural, political or economic forces; and it is women who sometimes feel they must relinquish their birth child in order to protect that child. It is also predominantly women who choose or agree to take on the work of mothering another woman's child as her own. And it is primarily women, adopted as infants or children, and birth mothers, who have created networks across North America, Europe, Australia and New Zealand that support adoptees and birth mothers as they search for one another. And finally, women are at the fore lobbying for legislation that will enable all adoptees access to their birth records.

This collection was created as a forum for women—birth mothers, adoptive mothers and adopted daughters—to come together to write about their varied experiences. As an adoptive mother, I wanted to place my autobiographical writing alongside other women's stories. When I write with other women in a writing-group setting, and then share my writing with them, I acknowledge the important stories of my life. As I listen to other women read, I hear a portion of my life in their stories. Suddenly, one woman's most personal account becomes a universal story. *The Adoption Reader* has the same effect: it weaves together personal essays, stories and narrative poems and offers a deeper understanding of motherhood while illustrating the spiritual, psychological, cultural, historical, race and class issues inherent in the adoption experience. These many voices and perspectives create a moving and groundbreaking collection full of many truths, much eloquence and courage.

More than thirty million people living in the United States are directly affected by adoption—whether as adoptees, birth mothers or as adoptive family members. This number continues to grow as, each year, approximately sixty thousand infants and children are legally adopted. About thirteen percent of these are international adoptions—involving children born in other countries who are then adopted by United States citizens.

Most international adoptions are closed or anonymous. However, in the last few years, the number of open domestic adoptions (adoptions in which birth mother or birth parents choose the child's adoptive parents and full identifying information is shared) and semi-open adoptions (adoptions in which both families are only given identifying information about each other) now outnumber closed adoptions.

The number of informally adopted children, children being raised by adults other than the child's birth parent or legally adoptive parent, is unknown. As of 1993, more than four hundred thousand children, living in group or foster homes within the Unites States, remained legally available for adoption. Many of these "waiting children," whose numbers have more than doubled over the past decade, are children who have been separated from parents who are abusive or mentally, physically or economically unable to protect and nurture them.

Between 1945 and 1965 most of the country's "waiting children" came from middle- and upper-class white families. Tens of thousands of white women found themselves forced to spend a period of time in maternity homes or were sent to another family's home because they were bearing a child "out of wedlock" or a child not fathered by their husband. Once they delivered, the girls or women were usually coerced into giving their infants to an agency or physican who would in turn offer the child to white adoptive parents. Anonymity of the birth mother and the receiving parents was often required by state laws.

African American unwed mothers during this same twenty-year period, described by feminist historian Rickie Solinger in *Wake Up Little Susie*, were excluded from white-only maternity homes. Black unmarried women or girls sometimes put their children up for adoption, but more often kept the babies, or, the babies were informally adopted by "other mothers"—aunts, grandmothers, friends and neighbors—so that extended families merged into other extended families, thus maintaining the historic practices of communal societies throughout Africa, Asia and North America. Shay Youngblood's rich and vivid stories included here are fictionalized accounts of her experience of being raised in an African-American community during the sixties by "some of the wisest women to see the light of day."

In this collection, many of the birth mothers describe their emotional responses to the oppressive circumstances around being single and pregnant, and others relate the psychological anguish of not knowing the destiny of their birth children. Several of the birth mothers write about their reunion with birth children or meeting their children's adopted families—often conveying a journey of acceptance, relief, unimaginable joy, and finally, closure.

The number of women left with no choice but to carry their unwanted pregnancies to full-term or forced to give up their newborn infants to anonymous adoptive families dropped dramatically after 1965; once birth control pills and the IUD were available, and abortion, under the 1973 U. S. Supreme Court Roe vs. Wade decision, became legal nationwide.

The adoptive mothers in this collection are in lifelong partnerships or marriages, while others are single. They are lesbian, bisexual and heterosexual—and some would describe themselves as too exhausted to think about relationships outside of their responsibilities to their children.

Not having nine months of physical pregnancy to enjoy or endure, many of the adoptive mothers here describe the months of administrative and emotional pregnancy as they, along with their partners, wait for their child to be born or to be "assigned to them" by an agency, lawyer or birth mother. Instead of the long-awaited contractions, there is the long-awaited telephone call.

Many of these adoptive mothers' essays, like traditional birth stories of mothers and their birth children, describe those unique first moments, those first days, those first years between child and mother. But few of their stories are simple and straightforward. Instead, these mothers' stories are filled with social workers, passports, state officials, probate courts, airports, wheelchairs, Hindu temples and endless papers tucked in and around the baby's birth or arrival. Several of the women here describe their lives as adoptive or foster mothers to children who have been abused, neglected or born with fetal alcohol syndrome. One contributor writes about how one mother in every lesbian adoptive family must become invisible in order to legally adopt children and about her ongoing concern that an unfriendly state court system could interfere with or destroy her family's well-being.

The adopted daughters here explore their struggle to know, accept or construct an identity that includes their birth roots—historical, biological and cultural. Some remind us that the reunion between an adoptee and her biological parent can bring a unique mixture of ecstasy, irony, and happiness as well as pain or poignant emptiness; shock when a connection that "should" be there, isn't: "'I'm really not the person you're looking for . . . Why is this so important to you? It's not the mother who bears you,' she said, 'but the woman who brings you up who counts.' That from my mother, too. Did she really believe it? Or was it a bitter, but necessary, rationalization for what she had done?" writes contributor Florence Fisher, a leader in today's adoptees' search movement. Other contributors express the love and deep connections they maintain with their adoptive parents, as they explore their personal birth roots.

The birth mothers, adoptive mothers and daughters in *The Adoption Reader* convey the complexity of adoption and illustrate the many ways in which adoption has always been and continues to be a part of the human experience. In the future, more women may decide to choose adoption over birth-giving in light of the world's overpopulation problems. "The most important thing that individual Sierra Club members can do is not to have more than two (birth) children," says Judith Kunofsky, chairperson of the Sierra Club's Population Campaign. This "two child or less" theme is echoed by Zero Population Growth, a national environmental organization that promotes the need for the United States to cut its current population in half during the coming generations by decreasing our birth rate from 2.0 children to 1.5 children per birth giver. Such a decrease will require women within the United States who want to become birth-givers to limit their births to two children, with the expectation that an equal number of women will choose to adopt or to remain child-free.

In spite of the fact that the United States has the highest birth rate of the industrialized world, medical professionals continue to encourage infertile middle-class and other privileged women to use private health insurance coverage, or spend tens of thousands of dollars on medical procedures to achieve fertility. On the other hand, poor women, receiving federal Medicaid health insurance coverage, are not allowed, under the Hyde Amendment, to use their federal insurance coverage to legally terminate an unwanted pregnancy. Thus private medical organizations, along with state and federal laws, encourage privileged women to have babies and at the same time make access to abortion difficult for poor women. Both policies, of course, serve to maintain or to increase the nation's high birth rate.

At the same time, numerous working-class and middle-class families and single adults who would like to adopt find it difficult or impossible to qualify as adoptive parents given most states' stringent regulations. These anti-adoption or "parental screening" policies as they are called by Harvard law professor Elizabeth Bartholet in her book *Family Bonds*, often include prohibitions against creating multi-racial families, and prohibitions against single adults, disabled adults, lesbian and gay families and lower-income families.

As we enter the twenty-first century, the notions around and definition of family are changing and evolving and adoption issues will continue to play a large part in women's lives. *The Adoption Reader* illustrates these issues and adds an important chapter, informed by personal experience, to a continuing and vital dialogue. I hope you will enjoy reading this collection as much as I have enjoyed the process of reading, selecting, editing and now sharing the words of so many creative, brave and good-spirited women and their families. My greatest hope is that this book will encourage an understanding of the powerful psychological, spiritual, cultural, economic and racial implications of women's adoption experiences. I also hope *The Adoption Reader* encourages more women to write out their life stories. Through writing, we can better know our selves, and our lives, as we create communities of women, communities of families and communities of cultures in our ever-changing world.

Susan Wadia-Ells
April 1995
Putney, Vermont

BIRTH MOTHERS

LORRAINE DUSKY

Family Reunions

Seventeen years have gone by since I first wrote for a magazine about the daughter I surrendered to adoption, and how the experience changed my life. The year was 1976, and my daughter was ten. I was a senior editor at *Town & Country* and, superficially, I had a good life. I had a job I liked, a wide circle of friends and a swell apartment in Manhattan. But if you had talked to me long enough, you would have discovered that my self-esteem hovered somewhere between low and abysmal.

I was a mother without a child. I was a mother who searched for her daughter's face in those of children at shopping malls, in Central Park, anywhere children her age might be. The world was a giant stage upon which, at any moment, our paths might cross, our lives intersect. But would I recognize her? That was the question. Improbable, of course. Almost certainly crazy. I've talked to enough women like myself to know that this is what we all do.

Six more years of a kind of living death would go by before I would find her. But find her I did. This story, then, has a happy ending, not only for me but also for my daughter, Jane, and her adoptive parents, her other mother and father. Except for clarity's sake, I don't call them *adoptive* parents, and they don't call me *birth* mother. That's the politically correct term among adoptive parents and social workers, but it repels me, reducing the woman who had the child to no more than a baby machine. Both terms—*adoptive parents, birth mother*—are far too limiting for what we are to Jane. I know that some of you would say that they are her real parents. But we are all her real parents. Before they could be her parents, I had to be her mother. And because I could not mother her, they did.

How did I find her? Through the "adoption underground"—not an agency but a loose-knit chain of people who will help you find the person you are seeking, whether you are the adopted individual or the parent. I had heard about the adoption underground the way slaves heard about their underground: word of mouth, all very hush-hush in order to attract as little attention as possible. Providing original birth and adoption records to an individual, except by court order, is illegal. In two states, Kansas and Alaska, adult adoptees can get their birth certificates, but all remaining records are sealed by law.

I knew the underground might help me, but I hesitated, for several years. My daughter was too young. Conventional wisdom said I should wait: Wait until she was eighteen, wait until she was twenty-one, wait until she was on her own. Then I kept reading about how, in going through adolescence and their teens, adoptees have a harder time than the rest of us in establishing a sense of identity: so many questions without answers, no sense of connectedness with the past.

In a 1971 position paper, the American Academy of Pediatrics had asserted that healthy individuals need to know not only who they are but who their ancestors were. How can you know where you're going if you don't know where you came from? The message I took from this was, maybe I should not wait. Maybe she needs me now. She was not yet sixteen. But maybe conventional wisdom was wrong.

So I went ahead, paid twelve hundred dollars and, several weeks later, with racing heart and the courage found in a stiff drink, on a Wednesday evening in November, I was dialing Madison, Wisconsin.

She answered—I guessed it was she—and I asked for Mary, her mother. When I told Mary who I was, we both cried. And when she asked my name and address and phone number, I couldn't figure out why, except to imagine that she might lodge some kind of complaint against me for invading her family's privacy. But that was not the case at all. She was levelheaded enough to be concerned that, in my state, I might lose my nerve and hang up. Jane—that's our daughter's name—had told her that she wanted to find me, and her mother had agreed to help however she could. But she'd had almost no information to go on. After we'd spoken for a few minutes, Jane's father, Wayne, got on the line, and I reassured him that I wasn't a crazy person who was going to try to steal their daughter away—how do you steal a fifteen-year-old, anyway?

And then they put Jane on the phone.

Even as I write this, eleven years later, that first moment of contact sears through me with all its poignancy intact. We were both somewhat tongue-tied. At her end, her parents were listening to her side of the conversation. At my end, my husband was writing out questions on the margin of a newspaper, because I was in too much of a fog to come up with my own.

The Chinese believe that an imaginary red thread connects people who are meant to be together, and that nothing can ever break that line—not time nor distance nor circumstance. Two people may not be parent and child, or even members of the same family, but if the red thread exists between them, they will come together, no matter what.

All the years of yearning, hoping and praying had come down to this: My daughter and I were talking on the telephone. She was alive. It seemed as if some part of me had been holding my breath, holding in the pain for nearly sixteen years, and now, at last, I could begin to let it out. I could breathe again.

We met a few days later at an airport, with strangers and her adoptive father looking on. There was her awkwardness at not wanting to hurt her father's feelings as he watched, my tears, our initial shyness. But within a month, she was visiting me and my husband at our home in the East. The visits quickly went from a few days to two weeks, then to whole summers.

That is not to say that it was always easy between us. We have had times—months on end—when we didn't communicate at all. She was angry because I didn't live up to her expectations; I became fed up with the guilt-inducing hostility she could radiate, when it suited her, during our visits. But I always knew—even if she didn't—that the break was only temporary, that we would again be close, that we would be mother and daughter, that the red thread couldn't be broken.

Jane had to sort out her feelings about being adopted—*why had I given her up?*—and I was so filled with remorse that our visits would exhaust me emotionally. I couldn't give enough, do enough, be enough. I always came up wanting. I would explain why I had given her up—I had written a whole book about it, in fact, how it happened in 1966, when I was young, single, shamed and without the financial resources to go it alone. She said she understood, and on some level I knew she did. But she still had a mountain of rage to dig out from under.

During her first stay with us, she and I decided to write a short play and act it out for my husband, his children and a close family friend. What did she want the play to be about? An adopted daughter who found her mother. Jane worked into our little drama a scene in which the daughter was able to tell the mother just how angry she was. When we actually acted out the vignette, Jane put her hands on my shoulders and began to shake me. "Why? *Why?*" she asked, her voice rising. I wasn't really bothered by the incident or surprised by her emotions: She was only fifteen, and she was struggling to sort out her feelings, whatever they might be, however painful it might be for us to confront them.

Feelings don't run on logic; they operate pretty much the way they want to. No matter how often or how well I might explain why she was put up for adoption, the question still hung in the air: Why didn't you love me enough to keep me anyway? Healing was going to take a long time.

Those visits might have been difficult, but neither she nor I was giving up; and I was learning how to be a mother, *her mother.* How strict or easygoing should I be, for instance? What hours did she keep at home, and what hours should she keep when she stayed with us? Did she have to let me know where she was? Or could she just be gone for most of the day and half the night? Did I have a right to get annoyed if we were expecting her for dinner and she didn't show up? Should I call around town to find her? Throughout all our conflicts ran one most important question: Was she testing me to see if I cared?

As if in confirmation, Jane evinced a great need for what felt like nonstop attention, particularly during the first five or six years. And I simply couldn't give it. She was always understanding when I closed the door to my office to work, writing at home as I do. But when I was done for the day, and I was ready for a drink with my husband or a half-hour jog or just some quiet de-compression time, she was waiting. Waiting for me to spend time with her, and her alone. And the greater her need, the more I would shrink back, feeling that nothing I could give her could possibly fill up that bottomless hole in her heart. Years passed, but still I was overwhelmed with guilt. And she was consumed with need.

Yet we didn't look back. When she was twenty-one, Jane came to live with us for a year. Now the rules of our house were even harder for her to accept. Like any twenty-one-year-old, she wanted to be a free agent. So we argued: over her curfew, smoking in the house, not tidying up after herself, whether or not she would listen to our advice and give therapy a chance.

But are those atypical arguments between any parent and child, when the child is a grownup or nearly so? No. I'd had these sorts of battles with my parents, and they were fierce. It is a part of growing up, because to grow up, you and your parents have to grow apart, and that road is always rocky. So the problems we faced that year had more to do with mother-daughter issues than "Why-was-I-adopted?" issues.

Sometimes, in exasperation—desperation?—I would call Jane's other parents, Mary and Wayne, and we would commiserate. We all wanted what was best for Jane. And there were no jealousies about who could best provide that. Whatever—or whoever—would work was what we were after. On one of those calls, Mary referred to Jane as "our daughter." Such simple words, such a gift to me. I can remember exactly where I was sitting and how the kitchen looked, just as I can recall where I was when I learned President Kennedy had been shot.

Together Mary, Wayne and I were doing what we could to help our daughter merge her past with her present, her heritage with her now very extended family. Because her other parents had opened their hearts to me, Jane wouldn't go through the emotional growing pains of becoming an adult with the additional burden of a great gap in her history. She would be someone who knew her heritage, and it would give her a story she could integrate into her identity and sense of connection with the world. "If the adoptee never finds his or her parents—or, at the very least, their names—he or she goes through life with an inability to develop intimacy, which can spread to other relationships," says psychiatrist and author Robert Jay Lifton. We had done what we could to ensure that would not happen to Jane.

I've dwelled on our difficulties, but I also want to tell about the good times: getting a Mother's Day card in the mail, and maybe a phone call during the day; buying her a pin-striped suit and knowing that I would have bought myself the exact same one if Loehmann's had another; calling her on her birthday and telling her I loved her and hearing the words back. Can I explain what it means to be able to call her on her birthday, after all the years, when April 5th was the bleakest of days? And then there are the simple pleasures that most mothers know over a lifetime, such as taking her to lunch, spending the day—the whole day—at Macy's, picking out a movie to rent because "it's our kind of movie," acting silly, even goofy, but knowing exactly why we are doing it. Such small incidents don't make interesting stories, but they are the stuff of dreams. They are what has transformed my life. Before there was despair; now there is a pillow on our bed she embroidered with a quote from Keats: "A thing of beauty. . . . " I'm not handy with needles and yarn; maybe she got that from my mother. The guilt and anger of our early days seem far removed today.

Jane and I are alike in so many ways, ways we are still discovering. We are both rabid liberals, both feminists at heart, and we both entertain a basic skepticism about authority. We can be moody one minute, silly the next. We have many of the same mannerisms, from a quick walk to an inability to snap the fingers of our left hands. We can't whistle, we sing off-key, we swear with the assurance of a truck driver. And sometimes we speak in a kind of short-hand that makes our years apart seem irrelevant. She looks like me—same body type, same ash-blonde hair—but I can see her father in her, too.

Jane never met him. It wasn't that she and I didn't try to make it happen; we did, and although he said he was willing, it was always "Maybe next time." He died before that day came.

She's twenty-seven now, married and the mother of a daughter herself. She lives in Madison, where she grew up, not far from her other family. She was here not long ago for five days with her husband and baby. I could hardly believe this was happening—that I would be able to know and love my daughter's daughter, as well as my own. And I could hardly believe that my story—which once seemed so common yet so tragic at the same time—has had a happy ending.

Her mother once said that things were better between her and Jane since Jane and I had found each other. Now there were no unknowns clouding their relationship, no wondering about what would happen if . . . because it had already happened. I don't think it's always been easy for Mary—she said that she was taken aback when she first saw how like me Jane was—but I hope that whatever fears she had were proved unfounded. Jane just happens to have a life that began with me and continued with Mary and Wayne and then again included me. It is her story—her full and complete history—and she has a right to it.

So does everyone. Because I am a player in the movement to open birth records for adult adoptees, I get mail and phone calls from women like myself and from adopted "children." Some are in their sixties and seventies; time is running out for them, and what they fear most is that they will die without learning their complete stories. Most of them will.

I've been writing back to these people and lobbying with them for change in the laws governing adoption confidentiality since Jane was five—more than twenty years ago—yet the laws have not budged in any real fashion. In the late seventies, the Supreme Court refused to hear a case dealing with whether sealed birth and adoption records should be opened. Historically, slaves have been the only other group of people similarly deprived of a full and complete knowledge of their heritage. The existing records on slaves date from their arrival in America; the records on adoptees are sealed by law. Slaves were denied knowledge of their heritage, separated from their kin without any thought of the effect it might have on them. A closed adoption realizes the same end.

As I write this, a bill that would open the records for adoptees at age twenty-one is under consideration in New Jersey. The fact that one of the bill's sponsors is an adoptive father with a thirteen-year-old daughter represents a dramatic shift from the past, when much of the legislation that closed adoption records was sponsored by adoptive parents. In New York in the thirties,

Governor Herbert H. Lehman was behind the legislation that sealed birth records in that state, and in 1980 the late Senator John Tower cast the vote that killed a provision that would have opened the records to all adoptees and natural mothers in the country. Both Lehman and Tower were adoptive fathers.

Regardless of how slowly the laws grind toward reform, however, the public's attitudes have changed. Private adoptions of infants are now rivaling agency adoptions, and most of the former are open adoptions in which everybody knows everybody right from the beginning. Given a choice, I would have chosen an open, and private, adoption. I would have insisted on choosing the parents. I might not have been wise enough to choose Mary and Wayne, but at least I would have made the decision about my daughter's future myself. In the 1960s, however, an agency adoption seemed to be all that was available to me, and with it came the awful, forced veil of secrecy. Such adoptions are grossly inhumane to the birth parents and the child, and have been ever since someone thought them up.

The sad part is that the open adoptions carried out today will not help the millions of parents who will never know their children, the millions of children who will never know their first parents, never even know what their stories are. How can this possibly be in the best interests of anybody—mother, father or child? How can it even be in the best interests of the adoptive parents?

As for Jane, someone once asked her if she would have had a happy life if I had not found her. She thought for a minute and then answered: "Yes," she said. "But not as happy."

JODY LANNEN BRADY

Talk of Babies

This is how it happened: A doctor dies. His children close out his files; my maiden name is on one of the files. The doctor's daughter gets my number from my mother's maid and calls me, not understanding how little I know. She asks: "Do you want the file?"

I am standing in the kitchen; my daughter tugs on my shirt sleeve, my son calls from the next room. Do I want the file? I want the file, and I want more than the file; I've been waiting twenty years for this phone call. I whisper into the phone: "Where's my baby?"

What does he know? What does he wonder? Does he wonder about me?

Does he have my cowlick on his hairline? Does he have my blue eyes or the brown eyes of his father, that boy from so long ago?

Did I give him to good people? Did he get his shots on time? Did someone make him eat breakfast in the morning?

Did he save money from a paper route to buy his first ten-speed? Did he go to his high school prom? Did they send him to college?

I got pregnant back when they still sent pregnant girls away. My father didn't speak to me; he made all the arrangements. He was a doctor and had offered, sensibly, to give me an abortion himself. I don't know how I felt about abortions; I might have even had one, except that the idea that my father was willing to kill his own grandchild was more than I could stand. And so he sent me away.

10

My mother did the explaining: "You're going to stay with Aunt Grace, up at Monmouth. No one has seen you in years, and they won't recognize you. You probably won't see anyone, anyway, but just call your aunt 'Grace.' She'll say you're a friend of the family, that your husband was drafted. Here's the ring. And your name is Beth Bridges."

The name was obviously my mother's idea. "Beth" was Elizabeth—my middle name—so I wouldn't feel like a stranger. And "Bridges" was her mother's maiden name, so I wouldn't feel as though the family had thrown me out. My father must have told my mother to come up with a name, and she probably spent hours deciding on what would suit us—my father and me. Anonymity for my father. Comfort for me.

There were no tears, no tirades of anger or remonstration. No interest in extracting a pound of flesh from the boy "who was responsible." If they had cried or gotten mad, it would have been easier. It would have been something that shocked them or at least surprised or disappointed them. But, as it was, my pregnancy came off as something they'd always expected of me. I was always letting them down one way or another, they seemed to be saying. This time was simply more inconvenient.

And so, without discussion, I was packed off to live with my aunt in Maine until "it was all over."

"Where's my baby?" I whispered into the phone the day the doctor's daughter called me.

The daughter was confused.

"I'm afraid I've made a mistake," the woman said. She repeated my maiden name.

"Where's my baby?" I asked again, louder this time.

A pause, and my heart stopped. Was the line dead? Had I only imagined the woman? But I felt the phone in my hand, and I heard the woman's breath over the line.

"But the babies are dead," she said suddenly. "I'm sorry. I don't understand. I only wanted to know if you wanted the file."

I hung up.

My daughter begged me to make her popcorn.

The woman called back. She began explaining—trying again: The doctor had died, they were returning his files or destroying the ones they couldn't return.

I cut through her words.

"Do you know who you're talking to?" I asked her.

She did.

"What are you saying?"

And again: the doctor's death, the file full of examinations, letters, adoption papers, death certificates.

I hung up.

My son sent something crashing in the other room. My daughter looked up at me, ready to cry in her brother's defense. I was aware that I should find out what had broken, but I slid into a chair and stared at my hands as they gripped the edge of the table.

"Does he know?" Aunt Grace asked me after I'd been with her a few days.

We were sitting on her front porch, moving slowly in the swing. I lifted my hands off my belly's swell to hold the hair off my neck. It was a hot day, but the steady breeze, coming in from the shore, kept us pleasantly cool.

"Does who know?" I asked her.

Aunt Grace looked down the street. She said something I couldn't hear. I had to ask her to say it again.

"The boy," she said and then turned to look straight at me. "Does the boy know you're going to have his baby?"

I sat back in the swing, and it moved sideways, banging the railing. Aunt Grace startled—her hands reached for the rail in front of her, ready to steady us, to prevent any accident. But the swing steadied itself, and I didn't upset it again. Did the boy know I was going to have his baby? He didn't—unless he had guessed the reason I had suddenly stopped seeing him and then dropped out of school a month and a half before the end of our senior year. And if he had guessed, why hadn't he done anything to find me, to ask if I needed any help? I hadn't thought about him. I hadn't known him well enough to consider him a way out, and I didn't like him well enough to miss him when I stopped seeing him.

"I never told him," I said.

Aunt Grace made a noise in the back of her throat. It was a noise she often made, not clearing her throat but close to that noise. It signaled neither disapproval nor agreement. It meant she was thinking and that I oughtn't say anything for a minute.

I felt the heat. I can feel it now, just thinking about it. Had the breeze stopped? I fanned myself with my hand and waited for my aunt to speak again.

It was a relief—finally—to talk to someone about the baby.

The doctor's daughter called back. My son ran in and answered the phone. Cautiously he handed me the phone, still waiting for a response to the crash he had caused in the living room. I patted his shoulder and then took the phone from him.

"Clean it up," I told him before I grunted a hello into the phone.

The woman must have realized that I hadn't known what the file contained.

"My father wrote your father. I have a copy of the letter. It's here in the file. I had to assume you knew."

"You're a sick woman," I told her because I could think of nothing else to say.

"Please," she implored.

"Please," my daughter said. "The popcorn."

My parents never spoke about the baby . . . about the babies—I had twins on the thirtieth of August. One, the first, came out stillborn. The nurse cried out when she saw the baby and tried to shield me from seeing him. The doctor said nothing; he knew of my situation and had made his disapproval known to me on every visit.

He had taken me on as a professional courtesy to my father, whom he had known at medical school. He allowed me to stay awake during the delivery—something not done back then—because, I am certain, he thought I deserved the pain. In the waiting room, in front of the other patients, he addressed me as "Mrs. Bridges." In the privacy of his waiting room, he called me "Miss Reardon," with a snide emphasis on the "Miss." And so, when he saw that my baby was born dead, he undoubtedly saw it as a form of divine justice. He moved the baby to a table beside me. The nurse quickly covered it with a sheet and came back to hold my hand. The doctor turned back to me, ready to deliver my placenta. What he delivered, instead, was a little, slippery baby boy.

That baby was more frightening than the first. The first was big and still. The second one waved his tiny, clenched fists. He was blue and bloody, and he called out in a pathetic wail.

The woman told me again about her father and the file. And then she told me how—"certainly, regretfully"—she felt she had to tell me that the child I had given away twenty-one years ago had died soon after I gave him up.

I hung up, this time not out of confusion. I believed the woman as well as I could believe anything. She knew my maiden name, she knew where I had stayed and she knew the name I had chosen for my son. I hung up because I was afraid of believing her. I hung up, but kept my hand on the receiver of the phone.

"Is that person going to call back again?" my daughter asked me. "Can't we make the popcorn now?"

"I'm hungry," my son yelled from down the hall.

"We are hungry, Mother," my daughter implored.

I unplugged the phone and made popcorn, carefully—oh, so carefully—moving step by step: oil coating the pan, the heat on medium-high, enough kernels to cover the bottom, quick shakes to coat the kernels, vigilance for the first pop.

Popcorn. Birthday cake. Packing school lunches: one sandwich, one fruit, one snack, one drink. Eating popsicles in the parking lot of the pool. Chocolate chip cookie dough. Flaming marshmallows held too closely to the coals.

I have cried over all the things I haven't gotten to share with him. I have cried over that child for twenty-one years. I have cried because I'm worried for him, and I have cried, knowing that he is the only one in this world who could chase away my loneliness.

On the thirtieth of August every year I spend the day alone. Without discussing it, my husband makes arrangements to free the day for me. He stays home from work with the children. He diverts errands and shopping his way. He wards off my employer. He has never known what to say all these years since I told him about Matthew, explaining my reluctance to have children. He has never spoken, but he has done his best to leave me room for Matthew.

It was he who first suggested I take a trip up to Monmouth and visit Aunt Grace, although she is in a nursing home and does not know who, if anyone, visits her. I think he hoped that visiting the place where Matthew was born would help. That talking to Aunt Grace, who had been with me while the twins were in my womb, would comfort me.

But it was only more silence. Aunt Grace didn't speak because she couldn't. My husband wouldn't talk about why I should go. My parents ignored me when I told them that I was going, and talked, instead, about the weather at the beach that time of year. No one has ever talked about Matthew. No one speculates, or sympathizes or offers advice. He exists only inside me and because there is no way to let him out, he has grown bigger inside me every year. I feel him more. I hear his thoughts. I see the world through his eyes.

When my son Peter was six years old, he begged me for a big brother. It was something he carried on about for weeks. My husband heard him once and yelled at him to be quiet and never to talk about a brother again; my husband thought he could spare me the pain of recalling my lost son. Peter never spoke of a brother in front of my husband again. It became our secret until he forgot.

I told Peter that he had a big brother who had to go away to live with another Mommy and Daddy who couldn't ever have any children of their own.

"How old's my brother?" Peter asked me.

"He's fifteen years old."

"When can I see him?" he asked.

"He's coming to see us sometime. I just don't know when," I said.

I hadn't realized, until then, that I had always assumed he was going to find me. I hadn't recognized my need for a fourth bedroom as preparation. I hadn't seen my labeling of family photo albums as anticipation. But I came to see that so much of my life since the day I held Matthew—for that was to be his name—had been waiting to see him again.

"How will he find us if he doesn't have our address?" Peter asked, ever practical, ever planning.

"I'll give him our address," I said.

"How will you give him our address if you don't have his?" Peter was exasperated with me. He exhaled a puff of breath, a perfect imitation of his father's impatient state.

I thought I would finally have someone to confide in, to speculate with. But when Peter saw through my assurances that he was going to get an older brother, he lost interest and pursued something more attainable: A few weeks of work on his father and he got a puppy.

I, on the other hand, was haunted by his questions. How *would* Matthew find me? I wrote a letter to the hospital where he was born. I received a brochure in the return mail: "The Rights of Natural Mothers." I had no "rights," it turned out, except the right to put a letter on file at the hospital, a letter saying that I wanted my son to be given the enclosed information should he inquire. Name. Current address. Age. Family medical history. Religious affiliation. Ethnic background. To the form provided me I attached a ten-page letter.

"Dear Matthew," it began. "You are fifteen years old now, almost a man."

I fixed my children popcorn the day the woman told me that my son had died so long ago. I fixed them popcorn, and then I sent them outside to play, and I tried to believe that Matthew had just been a sick baby, like his twin. That he'd lived a little longer but, like the other baby, never known anything more than sensations of comfort or discomfort. I thought: All these years I've missed something that never existed.

But I couldn't believe that. How could he have felt so real? Every birthday I've shared with him has been a lie? The letters I write to the hospital. Pictures sent to a ghost? Not even a ghost—just a figment of my imagination.

But he feels like flesh and blood. I can touch him if I can just reach out far enough. He's just around the corner. Matthew's out there, thinking of me—we are connected in our curiosity, our longing, our pain. We hate my father together—he is our villain. Matthew says to me: He wanted to kill me; he made you give me up.

I love Matthew as dearly as I love the two children here. I have suffered over his disappointments as much as theirs. I have worried over him as much. I've hoped for him as much. He's real. He's mine.

I finally told my husband tonight about the phone call.

"Go out, honey," he said.

Go out. Go cry. Go put up a headstone with the other one. Let it out. Let go. These are my husband's solutions.

I did not go out. I called the children in. They were out late because it is summer and they have no school now, but school is coming soon, for it is almost Matthew's birthday. I called the children in, and they came reluctantly.

"Brian's still out, and he's a year and a half younger than me," Peter complained.

I herded Peter into the shower and Kristen into the bath. I rubbed Kristen's slick body down with a towel and helped dress her and dry her hair. I threw Peter a towel and called to him to hurry.

"I shouldn't have to come in at the same time as her," Peter told me when he emerged from the bathroom. Steam clung to the room behind him.

"How can you stand to take such a hot shower in the summer?" I asked him. "Open the window in there."

Peter climbed up on my bed to have me read to him before bedtime; I hope he'll do it forever, but I know he won't. I read them a chapter of *Wind in the Willows*. Peter stopped me part-way to explain something to Kristen when she got confused. I didn't pay attention; I was feeling sleepy from the heat and from lying back and from the monotone of my own voice. Kristen roused me with a tickle, and I finished. We sang "Ash Grove." Usually at this point my husband chases Peter and Kristen to bed, but he had stayed away from me after I told him about the phone call. I could hear him in his office, working at the computer.

So I chased the children to their rooms myself. I tucked them in, and I kissed them—first Kristen and then Peter. I turned out all the lights, then I stood out in the hallway and waited until my eyes adjusted to the darkness. I looked in their rooms. I thought of the twin babies I had never tucked in bed, never sung to, never fed.

"Good night," I say to Kristen and Peter.

God bless and keep you, I say to the baby who died in my womb.

But I can't give Matthew to God. I can't let go of him. I might have saved him all those years ago if I had known to speak up for him. I might have hidden him from death.

I think of my father—of all the times he has spoken to me over the last twenty years, of all the opportunities he has had to tell me of Matthew's death.

I want to shout. I have something to tell my father—and all fathers, all mothers. I speak for Matthew when I tell them that children are not things to plan and arrange and manipulate. Children are pain: They are beauty and spite in the same breath; they are willful and needy; they are our life and our death, but they are never ours.

Who can say these things? Perhaps my father was simply no better at talking of babies than I am.

I shake my head and stumble toward bed. "Good night," I whisper to Peter and Kristen as I walk down the hallway. *"Good night,"* I say to Matthew as I crawl into my bed and dream him close.

KATHLEEN SCULLY DAVIS

A Love Story

The fragrant lilac hedge was several feet higher than our heads as we walked around the corner of Victoria and Portland streets on that precious Mother's Day. I was about to meet my first-born child, a daughter I'd given birth to twenty-three years before.

With me were my sister and soulmate, Mary Theresa, with whom I had marked this child's birthday every April, and my sixteen-year-old daughter, Tara, a dark-haired, dark-eyed clone of Mary. I, with my bright-red hair, was the odd one out of this trio.

Tara was crabby. That morning she'd brought me the newspaper and tea, but had snarled at the cat and seemed annoyed at life in general. I had said to her, "Honey, you're the one in this group who understands the concept of the loaves and the fishes. You know I won't take any love away from you to give to someone else. I'll just manufacture more. That's what moms do."

Tara, with sixteen years of practice in identifying and articulating an emotion the instant she has it, had answered with a dark frown, "I know that. But if you manufacture more love, I want it."

As the three of us rounded the corner onto Portland, I glanced at the three-story wedgwood-blue Victorian house that had been my first-born's adoptive home until her departure for graduate school. White trim and gables framed the stained glass windows, and predictably, the three-sided porch contained a porch swing. This was unquestionably the house of my own dreams, and certainly the perfect house for raising a family, this child of mine along with four siblings and three foster children. This blue heaven advertised "home."

My twenty-three-year-old daughter inside that blue Victorian had been one of the world's more wanted children. Her biological father, Angelo, had loved me more devotedly than anyone before, or possibly since. After only three months of dating, he'd given me an engagement and wedding ring set and asked me to marry him. He was quiet, gentle, unafraid to show his feelings and not ashamed to cry. In this land of stoic, unreadable Scandinavians, those were refreshing qualities. He was also never-married, Catholic and an ex-marine, credentials highly valued by suburban Catholic parents such as mine in the early 1960s.

But he was Mexican. To my folks, a "mixed marriage" meant marrying "out of the church." To marry out of one's race was simply unthinkable. It wasn't just the church, or my family. It was part of the mores of the times. The unwritten rule was to "stick with your own kind" and offer your counterpart virtue and inexperience at the altar. Many of us didn't meet that requirement, but the standard held.

Angelo and I were sexually active: already guilt-ridden over that "transgression," I did not want to compound it by adding the immorality of birth control. I was evidently still striving for the ideal. Though Angelo was also Catholic, he did not understand how making love could be a sin.

We knew I was pregnant before I missed the first period, and intuitively, so did my mother. I was twenty-one years old, certainly not a child, and the logical action would have been to marry the father of my baby since I was already wearing his engagement ring. But I was scared, ashamed and in a serious battle with my lifelong demon, depression. Angelo, on the other hand, was overjoyed and solicitous to my every need. He was ready to plan a wedding and shop for a place to live.

I told my mother I thought I "had to get married," a quaint euphemism of the time that would mean little to a young woman today. In 1962, there were limited phrases and concepts to describe an "indelicate situation." Mom was concerned and caring but uncertain that Angelo was the man for me because I'd spent years in a relationship with my high-school sweetheart and only four months with Angelo. Mom said I didn't "have" to marry him. She'd said we'd work it out. What she didn't say—what didn't have to be said—was that if I did not marry my baby's father, the child would automatically be placed for adoption. There were only two choices: I could marry and keep the child, or I could remain unmarried and give up the baby for adoption, a baby that would be considered of "mixed-race." Finding an adoptive home for my baby might be problematic, even impossible. I agonized over the decision. I was sick more than I was well. I hardly knew this man. There was still a spot in my heart for my high-school sweetheart. Marriage was unquestionably "forever." If I married Angelo, would the marriage work, given my reservations and the cultural gap? His mother grew her own chilis!! I didn't even know what a chili was! I had been raised on potatoes, for heaven's sake! Would our families reject each other? Would they reject the baby? What if we married and the marriage didn't work? Divorce was not a possibility. And even in the remote chance of a divorce, the child would not have two parents: the whole reason for placing the child for adoption would be to ensure a "two-parent family," and of course, all the "advantages."

The pressure from my family to not marry Angelo and place the baby was intense; to them, marrying this man was out of the question. Even as I was succumbing to the pressure from my family, this man held to his adamant belief that we could overcome obstacles. But, he was one person, and my family was barraging me from all sides. It took until I was halfway through the pregnancy, but I decided against the marriage.

Angelo's very large extended family was enraged. Angelo had no clear idea why, if I wasn't going to keep the child, I wouldn't let him keep it. Who ever heard of giving away babies? In the Mexican community there is *always* a place for a baby. Where did babies go who were given away? To an orphanage? He was incredulous at the thought. Everyone in his family, especially his mother, would take care of the child. He simply could not comprehend my "logic."

So I sent long, tedious letters of explanation to him about the Natural Order of Things, having no idea whatsoever that it might not be a universal order, that it might have been true for only a small, white, suburban, notoriously unbending group of people. We were under the impression that a child should have two parents, a mother and a father. At age twenty-one, I had never heard of keeping a child without being married. Only widows did that.

My painful decision was made. My baby would have two parents. Two adoptive parents. I was sent away, of course. A pregnant daughter wasn't allowed to stay at home, even to serve as an example to other children in the household. My pregnancy, like millions of others before mine, was to be a secret. I was supposed to be sorely ashamed. I was a failure at the only thing that mattered: being a good girl.

The strangers who gave me a home that bitterly cold winter did not at any time refer to the pregnancy. I, however, was consumed by it. When I was bathing, I would watch my stomach as it moved above the bubbles. I was so in love with the little legs and arms and feet. If this baby was a girl, could I go through with the adoption? Maybe not. Perhaps I shouldn't know if it was a girl or a boy. Boys need dads. I could probably surrender a boy. But a girl? Maybe I could raise a daughter myself. Then, one day, I suddenly found myself in hard, heavy labor.

I had made several requests of the doctor and the social worker: Please render me completely unconscious. Don't let me hear the baby cry, and don't tell me anything, particularly the baby's sex. I wanted a guarantee of instant placement into the adoptive home, and that only the adoptive parents would be allowed to name the child. In my soul I thought she was a girl and had named her Theresa, after my sister. The doctor honored my requests. The agency staff honored nothing. They told me I had given birth to a daughter, and they named her.

As my sister, my young daughter and I approached the steps of the blue Victorian house, I had to instruct myself to exhale. I was a walking bundle of nerve endings. I stepped up first. Behind me, Tara, knowing from photos her new sister would be dark-haired, said to my sister, "Let's let her guess which of you is the real mom!"

The door swung open, and one of the world's most remarkable adoptive mothers threw both arms wide and said, "Welcome to our home!" I fell into her open arms.

Pat has evidently always been remarkable. She had been a public health nurse when she married and began her family. But after giving birth to two children, she was unable to carry any other pregnancies to term, a source of extreme disappointment to her, as a large family had been her lifelong dream. Aware of all the unwanted pregnancies, then as now, Pat wept over the irony that she and her husband wanted a large family and shared a lifestyle that could accommodate one, yet were unable to have more children. Finally, because she is a practical, sensible woman, she went to Catholic Charities to apply for adoption.

Susan was the family's first adopted child. Of partially Mexican descent, she had been placed with them some months before my baby was born. The adoption laws, in the state, at that time, stated that an adoption in a family had to be final before another could be begun. Though Pat and her husband had spoken for my baby, Susan's adoption wouldn't be final for several months; consequently, my newborn was placed in a foster home. Pat pleaded with the agency to allow her to name and baptize the baby, unaware that I had also insisted on this, but because of the archaic closed adoption laws of the time, she wasn't even allowed to see or hold her.

Pat brought my baby to her home in November and shortly thereafter took her to the cathedral where she was baptized Mary Alice. Entries into Mary's baby book characterize her as "sweet, placid, maybe lazy, but with a bit of a temper." She was exceptionally beautiful, with larger-than-life brown eyes. She was good-natured and easy to raise. Pat and her husband adopted one more child after Mary, a son of Spanish descent whom they named Karl.

At that time in her life, Pat's husband began to be absent from home more and more. She could see the clear possibility of being alone with five children, so she went back to school for her master's degree in nursing.

Eventually, Pat and her husband divorced and she entered her "hungry years." On the other side of town, I, who had married and divorced my high-school sweetheart, was walking the same austere path with my two other children. Both Pat and I were extending the milk by adding powdered milk, and when there was no milk, putting water in the cereal. We managed, as poor women have always done, and somehow the kids did not feel deprived.

Pat told me later she often thought how ironic it was that three women had given their children to her, presumably so those children would have a good home with two parents. In fact, all five children were living in a single-parent home. She never had a minute of doubt she could handle the situation, yet she was glad the birth mothers didn't know what had happened to their babies. Each year when the adoptive children celebrated their birthdays, Pat reminded each of them that another mother out there somewhere was also remembering the day.

Pat managed the three-story house, grew and maintained a large garden and participated in parental activities at school while attending graduate school full time. She also began dating the man the children called "Mr. B."

I stepped forward and wrapped my arms around this woman, and she held me for a long moment. This was my daughter's mother. We whispered, "Thank you, thank you," to each other. Then, as now, I could not love her more than if she were my own sister.

Pat released me and introduced her daughter Jody, standing next to her. Petite and poised, she seemed to be loving this. Tara, behind me, was so agitated that she was oscillating. Since her brother had gone to live with his father, Tara had become accustomed to being an only child. Though she had known of her sister's existence for years, the reality that Mary Alice and possibly the rest of her family were to become a part of our lives was a definite cloud on Tara's horizon. Jody, however, was clearly curious and glad to meet us.

I looked into the shadows of the door and my eyes came to rest on Louie ("Mr. B"), Pat's second husband. A large, tall man, he nearly filled the doorway. Louie had married Pat after her divorce and his first wife's grueling death, and when Mary was twelve, had adopted all five of Pat's kids, "just in time for braces and college." Subsequently, Pat and Louie took in three foster children and offered their home to numerous others.

Louie had agreed to send Mary a ticket home from graduate school for this meeting, but his heart was clearly not in it. He was visibly apprehensive and his light blue eyes were misting over.

About a month before, the telephone wires had been alive with conversation between Mary Alice and me, Pat and me, and Mary and Pat. Then Louie had called me to say he wanted to be part of the group. It seemed that, for Pat, my presence in Mary's life was just one more person to love her child. But to Louie, perhaps, I was one more person for Mary to love.

Likely Louie was feeling somewhat as Tara felt, that there was a new person here who was going to change the configuration, and there was no way to control it. Tara had said earlier, "This Mary is no one in particular to me. She's just another person in the universe." Underneath that bravado was terror. And there I was, another person in Louie's universe. Unknown quantities. The middle-aged man, and my sixteen-year-old, shared an uncertainty bordering on panic. The grown man and the teenager were failing to do what they both usually relied on under pressure: Keep it light, keep everyone laughing.

Louie had been husband to Pat and dad to eight kids, but he is a complex man and has a separate relationship with each family member: Now he wanted his own relationship with me as well. He had advised Pat not to "push" Mary Alice into meeting me, knowing she would accommodate Pat's requests. But a small part of him didn't want to lose Mary, or even share her. He looked directly at me with his heart in his blue eyes.

"Come on, Mary," Pat said into the shaded room, "Stop hiding!" The rest of the family was stacking up behind Louie. Mary came around from behind Louie, timidly, hesitantly smiling, but anxious. She was flanked by her primary support system, her entire family. I could see she was much more beautiful than the pictures she had sent me. Somewhat over five feet tall, round and quite dark-complected, she had a crop of thick, dark, wavy hair and huge dark eyes. Those were my teeth in her smile, and they were translucent.

The look on her face was a combination of curiosity and stage fright. It was as if she were thinking, "How did this happen? I was just going along living my life, being totally content with my existing family. I wasn't even all that curious, not like Susan was curious, about my biological mother, and now here she is on my doorstep. I feel nauseous. How do we act? What do we do? What if I don't like her? What if she doesn't like me? What if I throw up in her face? Maybe I could cancel this whole deal. Maybe I could wish myself to disappear. What if there had been open adoption when I was born? I'd have had to contend with this total stranger all this time. She is no one to me anyway, just another person in the universe."

Her initial letter to me the previous January had been the very letter that every woman who has given up her child wants to receive. She had told me that she'd had a wonderful life, that she'd been educated at St. Catherine's College, where she had majored in Spanish. She'd been to Mexico and to Spain. She had the greatest parents anyone could ever ask for, and she had said, "Thank you for letting me have this kind of life." The letter went on to say she couldn't imagine any other kind of life, but that she was a little curious: Did she have any birth brothers or sisters? Why was she finding white hairs in her head at twenty-three? Did anyone else have a weight problem?

She had assumed she wasn't wanted at the time of her birth—she told me later that that is a common assumption for adopted kids. But she had a rich life, a wonderful mom and an adoring grandmother. She didn't have any need for another mother-figure. Plus she had this great dad who was threatened by this bio-woman, and nothing on earth was worth making him this nervous. What else could she want? So why was she standing here looking at a total stranger who didn't really have all that much connection to her life? Someone who *gave her away?* As difficult as my decision was to place her for adoption, her decision to meet me was equally difficult, and written all over her face.

I was riveted to the ground. This was a fully grown woman of breathtaking physical beauty and with the sweetest smile on earth, and she was stepping up to me in stop-motion.

She came within arm's range. I could hardly move. As most mothers do at the moment of birth, I touched her face, her hair, put my hands on her shoulders for the first time and fell instantly and completely in love with her. I said, "You're beautiful." I touched her again, and she continued her dazzling smile. I said, "I never even touched you," and the realization struck. This is my daughter as much as if I'd been there for the first step, the first lost tooth, the first period. This priceless child of God, with her mom behind me and her dad in front of me, was my daughter. A sacred moment, as the moment of birth always is.

We hugged softly. Then tightly. She scrutinized me, and then Tara. Finally she said to us both, "Well, I guess the weight problem doesn't come from you!" But then my bodacious sister Mary Theresa stepped up to her, and she said, "Well, maybe."

Suddenly there was chaos. Everyone was being introduced to everyone else, her brothers and sisters, and her two gorgeous nephews. Louie was offering coffee, mimosa, jokes that spoke of relief and joy, jokes for which the kids assured him he needed to get "some new lines." It was noisy and confusing.

Mary Alice asked me if I would like to tour the blue Victorian. So she walked us, her biological mother and aunt and half-sister, through her childhood in that house. She was soft and gentle, poised and sweet beyond words. Despite the shattering intensity of the hour, she maintained a calm demeanor.

I felt a quarter-century of the shackles of agnosticism release in my soul. Surely, this is blessing. This is grace. This is reconciliation. The cultural sanctions were dumb, the laws of the church and the state were cruel. Maybe closed adoption is unhealthy, but this much I knew that day, and I know it as I write: That woman/child/baby belonged to Pat and Louie, to that house, to that life. It was exactly as it was meant to be. I had served as a surrogate mother for Pat: This child was meant to be with them. I don't understand it, or why it had to be so stupidly painful, but it was right. I felt surrounded by spirit. It was a consecrated moment. Resenting the rules and balking at fate the whole way, nevertheless, I had done something absolutely wonderful.

We sat down for brunch in the elegant dining room. Louie was obviously overcome with emotion yet not prepared to cry in front of all of us: He gave grace and we began to eat and to become acquainted. Tara, awed by the house and the wonderful mom and dad, to say nothing of Mary's beautiful younger brother, Karl, wondered aloud if it was too late for her to be adopted by the family! (She liked not being related to Karl, however!) I turned to my new daughter and gave her the engagement ring from her biological father that I'd worn when she was born and had worn as a pinky ring since.

Mary now wears that ring as a wedding ring since her marriage. Her family and I have an ongoing relationship, one that allowed me to attend her wedding, fulfilling a lifelong dream for me. I was inadvertently the main mother of the bride that day because Pat was in the hospital for emergency surgery.

Mary and her husband Mark and Pat and Louie have visited my parents in Arizona. My mother wept openly, and I heard her say for the first time, "We were never really sure we did the right thing." (*Now* she tells me! Go figure!) My family and I can now see what Mary Alice has always known: Pat and Louie and Mary, as well as the rest of the houseful of children and foster-children, belonged together.

Once Pat and I packed suitcases and drove up to Fargo, where Mary was beginning her career. She introduced us as "my moms." We are family. Since we've met, Pat has never referred to Mary Alice as other than "our daughter."

Now all eight children are gone from the blue Victorian, and the house has recently been sold. From a photograph of the house, I will cross-stitch a sampler for Mary. And Pat and Louie will be moving to my neighborhood, where we will continue our rich friendship, dear love for each other and staggering respect.

Sometimes, at odd moments, my heart becomes very full. There are so many adoptive parents aching for a child, and so many unplanned children, often born to women who have few resources. Currently, pregnant women experience extreme societal pressure to keep their babies, regardless of what is in the best interest of those babies. And there are laws that continue to pull babies from adoptive homes and put them back with biological parents, also despite what is best for the child. Babies are treated as property. Many children are not as lucky as my Mary Alice.

I am older now and wiser, and I know something I didn't know as a young woman: Love isn't enough. Love does *not* conquer all. Often, the greatest act of love is to give a child loving parents *and* some opportunities. Personal experience in our now blended family shows me clearly that loving parents don't need to be related by blood to their children. We are all children of God, or the universe, or life. Each new baby deserves the best home, and sometimes that isn't the home of the biological parents.

Kahil Gibran says, "Your children are not your children. They are the sons and daughters of Life's longing for itself." He also says, "All you have shall some day be given."

And I reply: *Everything we give comes back to us, a thousandfold.*

PRISCILLA T. NAGLE

This Is the Day We Give Babies Away

The Placement.

Here is one way to give away your baby.

First, you go see Mrs. Bronston at the Children's Home, three days out of the hospital. You're still so sore you can't sit up straight, and the chair is a hard wooden one so you have have to wear a smock over a skirt. Your hair looks awful. You didn't know you were seeing her in time to set it. You're feeling pushed. They're really rushing you, you think, because they're afraid you'll change your mind. And everybody there knows, "It's best for the baby" —that's all you hear. This is the most important impression you're ever going to have to make, because Mrs. Bronston chooses the parents for your baby. And you're not ready. There is no way you can feel "at your best."

You hate Mrs. Bronston, you hate her questions, and you're sitting there giving the wrong answers to most of them: "Do you want your baby to have a Catholic or Protestant home, or does it matter?" "Protestant." "Do you think your son should be placed in a home in which the father is in the professions?" (Because she knows you're very bright). "Oh yes, that would be very nice . . . " "And what are your plans, dear, for the immediate future?"

So you tell her something impressive, mention a career that shows how ambitious you are and how much you care about humanity; later you want to bite out your tongue because you mentioned a local university—now she'll probably send your baby off somewhere and definitely rule out a professor at the university because you might *find out*. Everyone is always worried you'll try to find out. It never occurs to you to mention age, and later you regret it. Mrs. Bronston is sitting there looking totally together, and you know how you look, and she is making a living out of finding a home for your baby. It's

27

supposed to be a nice thing to do. But it absolutely doesn't feel that way. And you hate her not only for that, but also because you have to sit there and be so nice to her, and try to get her to think highly of you . . .

Mrs. Bronston, I want my son to have a home with a lot of love and warmth and caring in it. Parents who are secure about themselves and can be open and intimate and very understanding and supportive about the differences in people—especially their children. Why didn't you say that? I want them to be able to play with, talk with and enjoy my son for who he is. To teach him by example how to live life. I don't care if they have a religion or not. Or even how much money they have, as long as they have enough for good food. I want their spirits to be in touch with a power for good, whatever that is.

Why didn't you say that? You weren't prepared. And that isn't what she needed to know to fill out the paper. You never forgive yourself for not thinking clearly there. Never. But for a long time, you think it's her you're not forgiving.

The Visit.

Next, if you request it, you go to the Children's Home to see your baby the morning before you sign the papers. Two of you go together to see your babies. You feel watched the whole time, and you are. Everyone around is watching you, but trying to be subtle about it. So they bring you your baby, who starts to cry just before your twenty minutes are up. You don't know if there is an actual time limit, but that's about the longest anyone ever stays there. You didn't know that he was still technically yours until that day, that you could have visited him all along—of course it's pretty obvious why no one has told you that. It could be too upsetting.

Anyway, now you're holding him. Memorize his features. Some little kid who lives there keeps talking to you. The other mother keeps talking to you. You wish they'd all shut up so you could really see and feel him. He doesn't seem to like you. He doesn't want to cuddle. Your hands are as cold as death. No wonder he doesn't like being held by you. Both babies start to cry (oh no, you didn't get to undress him and look at him all over); you walk over to the doorway that opens down a long, long hall where you can hear other babies. Some woman who seems nice, but harassed and uncomfortable, takes him from your arms and goes away.

This twenty-minute picture never leaves you. You always wonder if they hold them and give them loving back there, down that long hallway, while they're waiting to be born again . . .

You step outside and look to the treetops, where you always h ... solace. And suddenly the pain hits. Deep and unbearable. All you can think is, Who will show him the beauty? Who will show him? . . . You realize years later that that was the first time it had occurred to you that you might have something special to offer him that others did not. That maybe you had the right to him, after all, and that this was a terrible mistake. But those thoughts are so out of your experience that you can't respond to them. All you can do is feel the pain.

The Signing.

That afternoon is the paper signing. You go to the Children's Home shortly after lunch and walk into a room with a table in it and two ladies sitting to the side. Mrs. Bronston is sitting at the table. You are introduced to the two ladies, who are there as witnesses. Your social worker is with you. Everyone is looking very uncomfortable. You are trying to look poised and lovely (someone tells you later you were white as a sheet). You are trying to make everyone feel at ease and to treat them graciously, because it's obvious they don't want to be there and that they're just doing this for you and they know you hate it.

Mrs. Bronston has you read the paper, but first apologizes for the language, says it's just a necessary legality. You correct the spelling of your name and the name of your hometown. You sign a paper that says, "I hereby abandon and neglect my child, (his name), and request that he become a ward of the court. . . ." They all stand up and half smile. You say, "Thank you," though you're barely breathing, because you want everyone to think you're wonderful so they'll work very hard to find your son a wonderful home.

The Hearing.

You walk into a giant courtroom, with the social worker, Mrs. Smith, and the nurse, and you're thinking, *Oh my God, it's as big as a church!* And indeed, it feels like a funeral. Your mind is numb, your body is cold, your hands are so cold they have no feeling. There are other people there. Teenagers and parents, all looking glum. *Oh no, are they gonna do this in front of everybody?* But you can't get out the question loud enough for anyone to hear.

Finally, you see this room's only used as a waiting room, because way up in front at an elevated desk someone comes out and calls the next case.

So you sit. And wait. The judge comes out once and calls Mrs. Smith up to him and talks to her—something you can't quite understand, though you hear words echo against the walls.

It's time. They call you, though you never remember what they said. Did they say your whole name? Probably not, for no one has said your last name out loud since you arrived at the home.

The three of you go inside to a normal-sized courtroom. You're all dressed up in your brown suit, wanting to look as nice as possible, still wanting to impress everyone so they'll make sure your son gets an especially good home. There's a young man there, in the benches at the right. Who is he? The nurse and Mrs. Smith seat you between them in the second row, right in front of the judge's high desk. He speaks kindly, but there's an edge of anger you can hear quite clearly.

The judge introduces himself, then introduces the young lawyer over on the right. You stand, the lawyer stands, you swear to who you are, and to tell the truth. It's all outside of you somewhere. The only word that's repeating in your mind is "horrible." The only feeling is "hurry." There seems to be no air inside you. All your insides are frozen.

The young lawyer keeps saying things to you. Something is terribly wrong. He's saying, "Are you aware that this will no longer be your child? Do you promise before this court and these witnesses that you will never seek to find him, or any information regarding him, again, for as long as you live? If you understand and agree, please answer, 'Yes, I do so promise.' "

"Yes, I do so promise."

He goes on and on . . .

"Yes, I do so promise."

They keep asking you to speak up. There is nothing to push your voice out. A scream is starting. Deep inside of you. Something is dying there. Something wants out.

The judge: He's supposed to just declare whatever it is he declares. But he starts asking you questions. He tells someone later he wanted to be sure you knew what you were doing, that you didn't look as if you were sure of what was happening. "How long had you known the father of this child? Was he aware of your pregnancy, and did he offer to help? No? Why didn't you inform him?"

"He had stopped seeing me. He had already graduated and left, and I didn't know where to get in touch with him." You don't tell him that your mind helped you deny you were pregnant for five months. You don't tell him that you thought you had to go out and change the world with your intellect, but now that your baby is real to you, he's the only thing that matters, and it's too late because you've already set the wheels in motion. And nothing in your whole life has shown you that you have the right to what you want just because you want it when it might hurt others. Nothing in your life has prepared you to believe that you have anything to offer your son that is special enough to keep him from what everyone says is "the best thing for him."

What is he doing? You have to get out of there. You're starting to lose the numbness that's holding you in one piece. You're starting to lose control over the screams.

It gets worse. He declares, banging a gavel, something wrong and terrible. You hear as you are leaving, ". . . that (your son's name) is now a ward of this court, and that he is no longer your son." Something else declares to you as you are leaving, *I will never be happy again.*

Run. Run and scream—where is the door? Outside. Outside the door you can run because the screams are overtaking you. But outside, there is someone waiting for you, and there is no place to run . . .

The screams never die. They just get locked away, driving deeper inside you. You learn to unlock them sometimes, to keep them from growing stronger and destroying you. But they never die. You live your life, you learn to find love and beauty, again. You raise your other children, you bury a child, but this one is always alive, and you don't know where, and you don't know how.

And you learn that there are decisions that are not right or wrong, they are just decisions. But if they are not natural to your deepest being, they change you forever, and the problem remains unsolved. He is real. And, alive or dead, he never dies to you. He is out there somewhere . . . lost to you . . . as you are to him.

BETH BRANT

A Long Story

Dedicated to my great-grandmothers,
Eliza Powless and Catherine Brant

About 40 Indian children took the train at this depot for the Philadelphia
Indian School last Friday. They were accompanied by the government
agent, and seemed a bright looking lot.

— *The Northern Observer*
Massena, New York, July 20, 1892

I am only beginning to understand what it means for a mother to lose
a child.

— Anna Demeter, *Legal Kidnapping*

1890

It has been two days since they came and took the children away. My body is
greatly chilled. All our blankets have been used to bring me warmth. The
women keep the fire blazing. The men sit. They talk among themselves. We
are frightened by this sudden child-stealing. We signed papers, the agent
said. This gave them rights to take our babies. It is good for them, the agent
said. It will make them civilized, the agent said. I do not know *civilized*.

I hold myself tight in fear of flying apart in the air. The others try to feed
me. Can they feed a dead woman? I have stopped talking. When my mouth
opens, only air escapes. I have used up my sound screaming their names—
She Sees Deer! He Catches The Leaves! My eyes stare at the room, the walls
of scrubbed wood, the floor of dirt. I know there are people here, but I cannot see them. I see a darkness, like the lake at New Moon. Black, unmoving.
In the center, a picture of my son and daughter being lifted onto the train.
My daughter wearing the dark blue, heavy dress. All of the girls dressed alike.
Never have I seen such eyes! They burn into my head even now. My son.

His hair cut. Dressed as the white men, his arms and legs covered by cloth that made him sweat. His face, streaked with tears. So many children crying, screaming. The sun on our bodies, our heads. The train screeching like a crow, sounding like laughter. Smoke and dirt pumping out of the insides of the train. So many people. So many children. The women, standing as if in prayer, our hands lifted, reaching. The dust sifting down on our palms. Our palms making motions at the sky. Our fingers closing like the claws of the bear.

I see this now. The hair of my son held in my hands. I rub the strands, the heavy braids coming alive as the fire flares and casts a bright light on the black hair. They slip from my fingers and lie coiled on the ground. I see this. My husband picks up the braids, wraps them in cloth; he takes the pieces of our son away. He walks outside, the eyes of the people on him. I see this. He will find a bottle and drink with the men. Some of the women will join him. They will end the night by singing or crying. It is all the same. I see this. No sounds of children playing games and laughing. Even the dogs have ceased their noise. They lay outside each doorway, waiting. I hear this. The voices of children. They cry. They pray. They call me. *Nisten ha.* I hear this. *Nisten ha.**

1978

I am wakened by the dream. In the dream my daughter is dead. Her father is returning her body to me in pieces. He keeps her heart. I thought I screamed . . . *Patricia!* I sit up in bed, swallowing air as if for nourishment. The dream remains in the air. I rise to go to her room. Ellen tries to lead me back to bed, but I have to see her once again. I open her door. She is gone. The room empty, lonely. They said it was in her best interests. How can that be? She is only six, a baby who needs her mothers. She loves us. This has not happened. I will not believe this. Oh, God, I think I have died.

Night after night, Ellen holds me as I shake. Our sobs stifling the air in our room. We lie in our bed and try to give comfort. My mind can't think beyond last week when she left. I would have killed him if I'd had the chance! He took her hand and pulled her to the car. The look in his eyes of triumph. It was a contest to him, Patricia the prize. He will teach her to hate us. He will! I see her dear face. That face looking out of the back window of his car. Her mouth forming the words *Mommy, Mama.* Her dark braids tied with red yarn. Her front teeth missing. Her overalls with the yellow flower on the

---

*Mother

pocket, embroidered by Ellen's hands. So lovingly she sewed the yellow wool. Patricia waiting quietly until she was finished. Ellen promising to teach her designs—chain stitch, French knot, split stitch. How Patricia told everyone that Ellen made the flower just for her. So proud of her overalls.

I open the closet door. Almost everything is gone. A few things hang there limp, abandoned. I pull a blue dress from the hanger and take it back to my room. Ellen tries to take it from me, but I hold on, the soft blue cotton smelling of my daughter. How is it possible to feel such pain and live? "Ellen?!" She croons my name. "Mary, Mary, I love you." She sings me to sleep.

1890

The agent was here to deliver a letter. I screamed at him and sent curses his way. I threw dirt in his face as he mounted his horse. He thinks I'm a crazy woman and warns me, "You better settle down, Annie." What can they do to me? I am a crazy woman. This letter hurts my hand. It is written in their hateful language. It is evil, but there is a message for me.

I start the walk up the road to my brother. He works for the whites and understands their meanings. I think about my brother as I pull the shawl closer to my body. It is cold now. Soon there will be snow. The corn has been dried and hangs from our cabin, waiting to be used. The corn never changes. My brother is changed. He says that *I* have changed and bring shame to our clan. He says I should accept the fate. But I do not believe in the fate of child-stealing. There is evil here. There is much wrong in our village. My brother says I am a crazy woman because I howl at the sky every evening. He is a fool. I am calling the children. He says the people are becoming afraid of me because I talk to the air and laugh like the raven overhead. But I am talking to the children. They need to hear the sound of me. I laugh to cheer them. They cry for us.

This letter burns my hands. I hurry to my brother. He has taken the sign of the wolf from over the doorway. He pretends to be like those who hate us. He gets more and more like the child-stealers. His eyes move away from mine. He takes the letter from me and begins the reading of it. I am confused. This letter is from two strangers with the names Martha and Daniel. They say they are learning civilized ways. Daniel works in the fields, growing food for the school. Martha cooks and is being taught to sew aprons. She will be going to live with the schoolmaster's wife. She will be a live-in girl. What is a *live-in* girl? I shake my head. The words sound the same to me. I am afraid of Martha and Daniel, these strangers who know my name. My hands and arms are becoming numb.

I tear the letter from my brother's fingers. He stares at me, his eyes traitors in his face. He calls after me, "Annie! Annie!" That is not my name! I run to the road. That is not my name! There is no Martha! There is no Daniel! This is witch work. The paper burns and burns. At my cabin, I quickly dig a hole in the field. The earth is hard and cold, but I dig with my nails. I dig, my hands feeling weaker. I tear the paper and bury the scraps. As the earth drifts and settles, the names Martha and Daniel are covered. I look to the sky and find nothing but endless blue. My eyes are blinded by the color. I begin the howling.

1978

When I get home from work, there is a letter from Patricia. I make coffee and wait for Ellen, pacing the rooms of our apartment. My back is sore from the line, bending over and down, screwing the handles on the doors of the flashy cars moving by. My work protects me from questions, the guys making jokes at my expense. But some of them touch my shoulder lightly and briefly as a sign of understanding. The few women, eyes averted or smiling in sympathy. No one talks. There is no time to talk. No room to talk, the noise taking up all space and breath.

I carry the letter with me as I move from room to room. Finally I sit at the kitchen table, turning the paper around in my hands. Patricia's printing is large and uneven. The stamp has been glued on halfheartedly and is coming loose. Each time a letter arrives, I dread it, even as I long to hear from my child. I hear Ellen's key in the door. She walks into the kitchen, bringing the smell of the hospital with her. She comes toward me, her face set in new lines, her uniform crumpled and stained, her brown hair pulled back in an imitation of a French twist. She knows there is a letter. I kiss her and bring mugs of coffee to the table. We look at each other. She reaches for my hand, bringing it to her lips. Her hazel eyes are steady in her round face.

I open the letter. *Dear Mommy. I am fine. Daddy got me a new bike. My big teeth are coming in. We are going to see Grandma for my birthday. Daddy got me new shoes. Love, Patricia.* She doesn't ask about Ellen. I imagine her father standing over her, coaxing her, coaching her. The letter becomes ugly. I tear it in bits and scatter them out the window. The wind scoops the pieces into a tight fist before strewing them in the street. A car drives over the paper, shredding it to garbage and mud.

Ellen makes a garbled sound. "I'll leave. If it will make it better, I'll leave." I quickly hold her as the dusk moves into the room and covers us. "Don't leave. Don't leave." I feel her sturdy back shiver against my hands. She kisses my throat, and her arms tighten as we move closer. "Ah, Mary, I love you so much." As the tears threaten our eyes, the taste of salt is on our lips and tongues. We stare into ourselves, touching the place of pain, reaching past the fear, the guilt, the anger, the loneliness.

We go to our room. It is beautiful again. I am seeing it new. The sun is barely there. The colors of cream, brown, green mixing with the wood floor. The rug with its design of wild birds. The black ash basket glowing on the dresser, holding a bouquet of dried flowers bought at a vendor's stand. I remember the old woman, laughing and speaking rapidly in Polish as she wrapped the blossoms in newspaper. Ellen undresses me as I cry. My desire for her breaking through the heartbreak we share. She pulls the covers back, smoothing the white sheets, her hands repeating the gestures done at work. She guides me onto the cool material. I watch her remove the uniform of work. An aide to nurses. A healer of spirit.

She comes to me full in flesh. My hands are taken with the curves and soft roundness of her. She covers me with the beating of her heart. The rhythm steadies me. Heat is centering me. I am grounded by the peace between us. I smile at her face above me, round like a moon, her long hair loose and touching my breasts. I take her breast in my hand, bring it to my mouth, suck her as a woman—in desire, in faith. Our bodies join. Our hair braids together on the pillow. Brown, black, silver, catching the last light of the sun. We kiss, touch, move to our place of power. Her mouth, moving over my body, stopping at curves and swells of skin, kissing, removing pain. Closer, close, together, woven, my legs are heat, the center of my soul is speaking to her, I am sliding into her, her mouth is medicine, her heart is the earth, we are dancing with flying arms, I shout, I sing, I weep salty liquid, sweet and warm it coats her throat. This is my life. I love you, Ellen, I love you, Mary, I love, we love.

1891

The moon is full. The air is cold. This cold strikes at my flesh as I remove my clothes and set them on fire in the withered corn field. I cut my hair, the knife sawing through the heavy mass. I bring the sharp blade to my arms, legs and breasts. The blood trickles like small red rivers down my body. I feel nothing. I throw the tangled webs of my hair into the flames. The smell, like a burning animal, fills my nostrils. As the fire stretches to touch the stars, the people come out to watch me—the crazy woman. The ice in the air touches me.

They caught me as I tried to board the train and search for my babies. The white men tell my husband to watch me. I am dangerous. I laugh and laugh. My husband is good only for tipping bottles and swallowing anger. He looks at me, opening his mouth and making no sound. His eyes are dead. He wanders from the cabin and looks out on the corn. He whispers our names. He calls after the children. He is a dead man.

Where have they taken the children? I ask the question of each one who travels the road past our door. The women come, and we talk. We ask and ask. They say there is nothing we can do. The white man is like a ghost. He slips in and out where we cannot see. Even in our dreams he comes to take away our questions. He works magic that resists our medicine. This magic has made us weak. What is the secret about them? Why do they want our children? They sent the Blackrobes many years ago to teach us new magic. It was evil! They lied and tricked us. They spoke of gods who would forgive us if we believed as they do. They brought the rum with the cross. This god is ugly! He killed our masks. He killed our men. He sends the women screaming at the moon in terror. They want our power. They take our children to remove the inside of them. Our power. They steal our food, our sacred rattle, the stories, our names. What is left?

I am a crazy woman. I look to the fire that consumes my hair and see their faces. My daughter. My son. They still cry for me, though the sound grows fainter. The wind picks up their keening and brings it to me. The sound has bored into my brain. I begin howling. At night I dare not sleep. I fear the dreams. It is too terrible, the things that happen there. In my dream there is wind and blood moving as a stream. Red, dark blood in my dream. Rushing for our village. The blood moves faster. There are screams of wounded people. Animals are dead, thrown in the blood stream. There is nothing left. Only the air echoing nothing. Only the earth soaking up blood, spreading it in the four directions, becoming a thing there is no name for. I stand in the field watching the fire. The People watching me. We are waiting, but the answer is not clear yet. A crazy woman. That is what they call me.

1979

After taking a morning off work to see my lawyer, I come home, not caring if I call in. Not caring, for once, at the loss in pay. Not caring. My lawyer says there is nothing more we can do. I must wait. As if there has been something other than waiting. He has custody and calls the shots. We must wait and see how long it takes for him to get tired of being a mommy and a daddy. So, I wait.

I open the door to Patricia's room. Ellen and I keep it dusted and cleaned in case my baby will be allowed to visit us. The yellow and blue walls feel like a mockery. I walk to the windows, begin to systematically tear down the curtains. I slowly start to rip the cloth apart. I enjoy hearing the sounds of destruction. Faster, I tear the material into strips. What won't come apart with my hands, I pull at with my teeth. Looking for more to destroy, I gather the sheets and bedspread in my arms and wildly shred them to pieces. Grunting and sweating, I am pushed by rage and the searing wound in my soul. Like a wolf, caught in a trap, gnawing at her own leg to set herself free, I begin to beat my breasts to deaden the pain inside. A noise gathers in my throat and finds the way out. I begin a scream that turns to howling, then becomes hoarse choking. I want to take my fists, my strong fists, my brown fists, and smash the world until it bleeds. Bleeds! And all the judges in their flapping robes, and the fathers who look for revenge, are ground, ground into dust and disappear with the wind.

The word "lesbian." Lesbian. The word that makes them panic, makes them afraid, makes them destroy children. The word that dares them. Lesbian. *I am one.* Even for Patricia, even for her, *I will not cease to be!* As I kneel amidst the colorful scraps, Raggedy Anns smiling up at me, my chest gives a sigh. My heart slows to its normal speech. I feel the blood pumping outward to my veins, carrying nourishment and life. I strip the room naked. I close the door.

ARTEMIS OAKGROVE

Full Circle

My daughter, Cassandra, turned twenty-two recently. I haven't seen her since she was five-and-a-half years old, when I gave her up for adoption. I had hoped she would contact me when she became old enough to legally petition the adoption registry for information concerning my whereabouts. Every time I moved, which was often, I religiously provided the registry with my address and phone number. I spent many hours mulling over our possible conversations, explaining to her why I gave her up. I resolved to be completely honest with her if she asked me questions about her childhood. I have always believed she deserved the truth, as I remember and understand it.

For the first few years after her adoption was final, I couldn't watch TV programs or movies that had small children in them; it was too painful. Now my internal radar is permanently set on adoption stories: I'll stop whatever I'm doing to read a magazine article or watch a talk show focusing on adoption, hoping that maybe I'll gain a better understanding of adopted children's attitudes toward their biological mothers. I especially enjoy the programs that feature reunions of birth mothers and the children they gave up.

One such story appealed to me because the birth mother's concerns about her daughter's lifestyle were much like my own. I was relieved to hear I wasn't the only mother who worried that her daughter might be a religious fanatic or ultra-conservative. I have a fear that if Cassandra did reach out to me, my lifestyle might cause her to withdraw in disgust and shame.

She knows I'm a lesbian. I came out when she was nine months old, after I left her father. And I was always completely up front with the state agency that handled the adoption. The social workers knew I was queer, as did the couple who adopted her.

When Cassandra's twenty-first birthday approached, I got out the paperwork I'd been sent by the state registry when I first signed up several years ago. I reread the letter from the Colorado Department of Vital Statistics explaining the adopted child's rights and realized, for the first time, that my fantasy of Cassandra's finally being able to contact me now that she was of age, was the stuff of illusion, illusion I had created to protect myself. When I read the fine print on the adoption registry papers, I realized that Cassandra could have requested information on my whereabouts any time she'd wanted to, simply by having her adoptive parents sign a waiver giving their permission. It was time to get real with myself. Cassandra probably wasn't one of those adopted children burning with desire to find and connect with her birth mother.

During the past year I have begun to embrace the possibility that her healing process may never include contact with me. For fifteen years, I needed her twenty-first birthday to be the day she could instigate contact. That day came and went without much fanfare or, surprisingly, much pain. I understand the need to avoid contact with one's biological family. I haven't been in contact with my own family of origin for nearly twenty years. This is why I will always respect her boundaries and not try to locate her.

Cassandra has every right to be bitter, angry and in no way willing to be in contact with me. There is a lot of pain involved in being abandoned by one's mother. I know from experience.

I believe that my ability to function as a mother was doomed in the wilds of turn-of-the-century rural Colorado. My great grandmother, a religious fanatic, disdained physical contact with her children. One of her daughters, my grandmother, had one child, my mother. As a child, my mother was packed off to her father's parents to be raised until she was fifteen. When I was eight my mother abandoned me and my brother. My father was granted custody at a time when this was almost unheard of. He then left us with his parents for the next two years. Where he was during this time is a mystery to me.

I'm able to see that if my mother had had access to AL-ANON, recovery literature, effective medications and cognitive therapy, she might have been the one to break her family's patterns of neglect and abuse. But she didn't. Instead she managed to get through her non-working days in her fifties tract house by smoking cigarettes and watching television. She was clinically depressed and thoroughly resentful of her role as wife and mother. My guess is that she probably would have been a lot better off not marrying or having children.

I never bonded with my mother. Bonding with people does not come naturally to me. Even when my own daughter was first placed in my arms, I was afraid to hold her.

What I also know now was that I had and still have anorexia. When I was three months pregnant, I weighed 105 pounds (I'm five feet, seven inches tall). If her father did nothing else for Cassandra, beyond providing her with his creative genes, he made sure I had enough to eat during the pregnancy. Cassandra was a perfectly healthy baby with an adequate birth weight. But Cassandra's and my health went downhill from there. The very moment the pregnancy ended, the cycle of self-starvation began again. From that moment until she was given a new permanent home, Cassandra's growth wavered between failure-to-thrive and the lowest part of the growth curve.

As ill-equipped as I was for motherhood, I was even less equipped for single motherhood. A few months after my divorce, I became bedbound by clinical depression. One day I looked around and saw I had practically no food in my tiny one-room apartment; Cassandra was wallowing in dirty diapers and soaked bedclothes; there was curdled soy milk in her bottle, and I had zero energy. I needed help, and somehow I managed to ask for it. I called Children and Family Services. That same day, a very nice, non-judgmental young woman came to my home and, at my request, took Cassandra from me and placed her in foster care for the next several months. By the time she was returned to me, she was old enough to go to day care. I will always be extremely grateful for those day-care settings and the people with children Cassandra's age who took an interest in her well being. Those were the people who nurtured her by making certain she was fed, socialized, taught, supported and loved.

As a toddler and pre-schooler, Cassandra was a delightful, beautiful child. She also possessed a tremendous amount of compassion for me, although she openly hated my lifestyle. She didn't want to be a vegetarian; she hated being an only child and she was deeply disturbed by the volatile affairs I carried on with various women over the years. Cassandra, the pre-schooler, was lonely and sad, just like her mother.

When Cassandra was five, I heard my mother's voice while delivering a brutal belting to Cassandra's bare bottom. I stood up straight, dropped the belt, and looked around to see if my mother was in the room. It wasn't her. It was me. I was doing to this beautiful, innocent child what my mother had done to me. Something was wrong. Very wrong.

By the grace of some greater being, I was able to see that I was repeating my family history.

This wasn't what I wanted for her. If she stayed with me, her life would be hell. Although I couldn't undo the damage I'd already done and had allowed to be done to her, I could try to prevent further damage.

I called Children and Family Services to take Cassandra away for the second and final time. A friend who had been with me the day I gave Cassandra away told me what a courageous thing I'd done. That's what everybody still tells me: It was a courageous thing to do; most people wouldn't have had the guts to act on their child's behalf that way.

Yet, I have always thought giving Cassandra up was an act of cowardice. I think it takes real courage to stick it out as a parent. However, every woman I've spoken to about this experience has, without qualification, insisted that what I did was an act of love. They all say that the real cowardly thing would have been to continue to subject my daughter to my abuse and neglect, which could have only gotten worse. To act to save her from that, in hopes that she could go on to someone who genuinely wanted her and was able to raise her, was one of the hardest things a mother could do.

What I have continuously prayed and wished for more than anything else during the past sixteen years is that my precious, beautiful little girl was able to spend the rest of her childhood in a nurturing environment. Knowing that I'm mentally ill and that Cassandra had been neglected and abused, I am hopeful that her adoptive parents took extra care to give her the therapy and guidance she needed to begin to heal her wounds.

The cycle needed to stop. It was my wish that she would have plenty to eat, safety, security, siblings, happiness, support and belief in herself. I didn't want her to grow up to be antisocial, violent, self-hating, addicted, suicidal, desperate, frightened and unable to trust as I had.

I didn't want Cassandra to grow up literally bereft of parenting skills. She seemed, to me, like someone who might very well want to have a family and would enjoy doing so. Even as a four- and five-year-old, Cassandra was very social. She had a tremendous amount of love to give. But I had begun to kill off any chance she would have to provide love, support and nourishment for children she might have.

Although Cassandra was placed with a family through a closed adoption, I was still allowed to know some basic facts about the people who had chosen to adopt her. They had one birth child, a daughter, but were unable to have more biological children. They fell in love with Cassandra the minute they saw her. The father was an art professor, the mother an early childhood educator. I couldn't have hoped for more. I'm a novelist and artist; her father is a musician. Cassandra has little choice but to be a creative person given her gene pool.

Cassandra is luckier than I was at her age. When I was growing up, my art was never safe. I had to hide it deep down inside me to keep it from being destroyed by my family. What more could I have asked than for Cassandra to be raised in an environment where art was not only safe, but encouraged? I *have* to believe that her life has been many times better with these people than it would have been with me.

It's been one hundred years since my great-grandmother was Cassandra's age, busily establishing or continuing this sad history of maternal neglect and abuse toward her children. I doubt if anyone could imagine how badly I want my act of giving her up to be a detour around my family's unconscious repetition of failed motherhood. I don't really care if Cassandra ever understands what I did, or why I did it. As savage and painful as her early childhood was, it was much less so than mine.

As a child, I had a recurring dream about being left outside on the front lawn during a tornado. I knew my family was safe inside, but for some reason I hadn't been allowed to join them. Instead I had been left outside to fend for myself. In the dream, curled into a hole in the ground, I stuck my thumb up above ground level, and the tornado took it off. At some other point in this dream, I desperately looked for a specific house where a woman lived who wanted to rescue me. Somehow I could never reach that house.

Not long ago, I was able to finally reveal the contents of this dream to my therapist. Her take on it was that the thumb is my source of security and the tornado took that security away from me.

That dream symbolizes the utter despair I felt as a child. I have to believe there were adults around me, in the mid-fifties, who wanted to help me but didn't know how. I *wanted* to be rescued by an adult and never was.

It is my fervent wish and dream that Cassandra's adoptive parents are the people in that house I could never reach to be rescued. I want to believe that my determination to end this deadly cycle has worked. I am willing to tell Cassandra everything, if she ever asks. I won't blame her if she never does.

MINNIE BRUCE PRATT

All the Women Caught in Flaring Light

1.

A grey day, drenched, humid, the sun-
flowers bowed with rain. I walk aimless
to think about this poem. Clear water runs
as if in a streambed, middle of the alley,
a ripple over bricks and sandy residue,
for a few feet pristine as a little creek
in some bottomland, but then I corner
into the dumped trash, mattresses, a stew
of old clothes. I pull out a wooden fold-up
chair, red vinyl seat, useful for my room,
while water seeps into my shoes. A day to
be inside, cozy. Well, let's pick a room:

Imagine a big room of women doing anything,
playing cards, having a meeting, the rattle
of paper or coffee cups or chairs pushed back,
the loud and quiet murmur of their voices,
women leaning their heads together. If we
leaned in at the door and I said, *Those women
are mothers,* you wouldn't be surprised, except
at me for pointing out the obvious fact.

Women *are* mothers, aren't they? So obvious.
Say we walked around to 8th or 11th Street
to drop in on a roomful of women, smiling, intense,

playing pool, the green baize like moss. One
lights another's cigarette, oblique glance.
Others dance by twos under twirling silver moons
that rain light down in glittering drops.
If I said in your ear, through metallic guitars,
These women are mothers, you wouldn't believe me,
would you? Not really, not even if you had come
to be one of the women in that room. You'd say:
Well, maybe, one or two, a few. It's what we say.

Here, we hardly call our children's names out loud.
We've lost them once, or fear we may. We're careful
what we say. In the clanging silence, pain falls
on our hearts, year in and out, like water cutting
a groove in stone, seeking a channel, a way out,
pain running like water through the glittering room.

2.

I often think of a poem as a door that opens
into a room where I want to go. But to go in

here is to enter where my own suffering exists
as an almost unheard low note in the music,
amplified, almost unbearable, by the presence
of us all, reverberant pain, circular, endless,

which we speak of hardly at all, unless a woman
in the dim privacy tells me a story of her child
lost, now or twenty years ago, her words sliding
like a snapshot out of her billfold, faded outline
glanced at and away from, the story elliptic, oblique
to avoid the dangers of grief. The flashes of story
brilliant and grim as strobe lights in the dark,
the dance shown as grimace, head thrown back in pain.

Edie's hands, tendons tense as wire, spread, beseeched,
how she'd raised them, seven years, and now not even
a visit, Martha said she'd never see the baby again,
her skinny brown arms folded against her flat breasts,
flat-assed in blue jeans, a dyke looking hard as a hammer:
And who would call her a mother?

                                        Or tall pale Connie,
rainbow skirts twirling, her sailing-away plans, islands,
women plaiting straw with shells: Who would have known
until the night, head down on my shoulder, she cried out
for her children shoved behind the father, shadows
who heard him curse her from the door, hell's fire
as she waited for them in the shriveled yard?

All the women caught in flaring light, glimpsed
in mystery: The red-lipped, red-fingertipped woman
who dances by, sparkling like fire, is she here on the sly,
four girls and a husband she'll never leave from fear?
The butch in black denim, elegant as ashes, her son
perhaps sent back, a winter of no heat, a woman's salary.
The quiet woman drinking gin, thinking of being sixteen,
the baby wrinkled as wet clothes, seen once, never again.

Loud music, hard to talk, and we're careful what we say.
A few words, some gesture of our hands, some bit of story
cryptic as the mark gleaming on our hands, the ink
tattoo, the sign that admits us to this room, iridescent
in certain kinds of light, then vanishing, invisible.

3.

If suffering were no more than a song's refrain
played through four times with its sad lyric,
only half-heard in the noisy room, then done with,
I could write the poem I imagined: All the women
here see their lost children come into the dim room,
the lights brighten, we are in the happy ending,
no more hiding, we are ourselves and they are here
with us, a reconciliation, a commotion of voices.

I've seen it happen. I have stories from Carla,
Wanda. I have my own: the hammering at authority,
the years of driving round and round for a glimpse,
for anything, and finally the child, big, awkward,
comes with you, to walk somewhere arm in arm.

But things have been done to us that can never be
undone. The woman in the corner smiling at friends,

the one with black hair glinting white, remembers
the brown baby girl's weight relaxed into her lap,
the bottle in her right hand, cigarette in her left,
the older blonde girl pressed tense at her shoulder,
the waves' slap on the rowboat, the way she squinted
as the other woman, her lover, took some snapshots,
the baby sucking and grunting rhythmic as the water.

The brown-eyed baby who flirted before she talked,
taken and sent away twenty years ago, no recourse,
to a tidy man-and-wife to serve as daughter.
If she stood in the door, the woman would not know her,
and the child would have no memory of the woman,
not of lying on her knees nor at her breast, leaving
a hidden mark, pain grooved and etched on the heart.

The woman's told her friends about the baby. They
keep forgetting. Her story drifts away like smoke,
like vague words in a song, a paper scrap in the water.
When they talk about mothers, they never think of her.

No easy ending to this pain. At midnight we go home
to silent houses, or perhaps to clamorous rooms full
of those who are now our family. Perhaps we sit alone,
heavy with the past, and there are tears running bitter
and steady as rain in the night. Mostly we just go on.

ROBYN FLATLEY

My Son

Hi, I think we may be related," he said.

"Oh, my God . . ." I couldn't breathe. He had not been killed in the Gulf War as I had feared. He was alive as I had hoped. For the last few weeks I had felt him coming closer. It was almost as if he had been taking form right before my eyes. I wasn't crazy; here he was on the phone with me.

We talked for six hours after twenty-six years of silence. With each new topic he quelled my fears of his being a skinhead, or a right-wing fanatic, or someone who hated women. All the years of asking young men when their birthdays were could stop, searching for his face in a crowd could stop. He was not bitter about my giving him up. I felt young again, and all the old urges I had had at eighteen were suddenly reactivated: I wanted to go out and get drunk, have millions of boyfriends again, be wild and mindless. I wanted to celebrate. He was sweet, funny, kind, intelligent and supportive. He was the kind of man I could fall madly in love with.

"Your voice sounds so young," he said.

"I'm only nineteen years older than you."

We talked about our parents and how they were similar: His father was a lawyer, so was mine. How our families were Irish and proud of it and how we were both the second youngest in our families. We seemed more like brother and sister than mother and son.

"I want to ask you about my biological father at some point," he said. I felt a flash of anger that the man who denied he had gotten me pregnant would get any of this precious attention.

"Sure, we'll talk about him later," I said.

"My parents don't want to meet you," he said, "but they did want me to say

48

'thank you.' My father cried when I asked him to sign the release form. I didn't want to hurt him, so I withdrew my request, but a week later he consented. He did ask that I see you only once, then never again."

"Will you do that? Will I see you only once?" I whispered. My heart was pounding as he replied.

"No," he answered quietly.

That week he called me every night. We talked politics, religion, sex and relationships. His intimate sharing was somehow erotic. He sounded as wild as I had been at his age. My parents and sisters called nightly, and I rejoiced with my boyfriend, Paul, and with friends. We set the date to meet. He would spend one night. I was barely touching ground. My son was coming home.

It was a rainy Saturday afternoon when we saw his car pull up. Paul greeted him at the door while I waited. He rushed into the living room. All the years of wondering who he was, and now my answers took the form of a tall, handsome man with a face that looked like mine but much younger. He had soft brown eyes, so different from my baby blues, and in his trembling hands he held a huge bouquet of flowers. I let them tumble to the floor as I fell into his arms. My body shook with recognition, and my uterus went wild, contracting into spasms. I had become eighteen years old again. But my baby was too big to cuddle and too old to breast-feed. He was a twenty-six-year-old man; I wanted my newborn baby back.

Later that evening, through the drizzling rain and ink-blue twilight, we walked to the center of the Hinsdale Bridge.

"I feel dizzy, like I'm in love with you," I said shivering, holding tight to his warm arm. I yearned to embrace him.

"You know, this is confusing for us both. I will never make love with you; it's against my beliefs," he said. He was dead serious.

I felt cheated and relieved. I wanted him inside of me and the only way I could have that again was to have this man. I cried as the rain bathed my face.

"I just don't know how to relate to you! I want to go out and get drunk, and I stopped drinking over ten years ago. I just don't know who I am right now." I felt torn apart by all the eighteen-year-old desires I thought I had long ago left behind.

The river mist encircled us. We turned back to the apartment.

Later that night, after Paul and his own son had gone to bed, Shawn and I pored over his baby pictures. He had brought along a videotape of all the Christmases I had missed, and with my encouragement he pushed it into the VCR. A large lump grew in my throat as I watched Shawn animatedly talk about the fun and the special gifts of those years. The grief for having missed his childhood rose into my mouth, bitter and sour. I began to cry.

"Oh, God, the back of your head feels just like mine!" he said, as his hand cradled my head.

I wept harder.

"My childhood was great," he said. "I was loved. It was the right thing to do . . . giving me up." He was defending my choice. "I would have been so angry being raised without a father."

I blocked my ears. "It makes me furious that I didn't keep you!" I raged, my lips twisted in pain. I remembered why I had given him up. My mother, a manic-depressive, had had her first breakdown shortly after my birth and continued to be hospitalized every two years of my life. She admitted to me recently that she had not been able to love me. I felt relieved to know the truth. I had watched her love my baby sister and then turn to me with a pinched look on her face. Before my unwanted pregnancy, I had made a pact with myself not to have any children. Between my mother's lack of love and her illness, I had had grave doubts about my own ability to love and rear a child. I just couldn't pass on these painful emotional and genetic problems to another generation.

Those fears felt flawed to me now as I studied the shimmering image of my baby on the television screen. I wanted him in my arms, this precious little boy. Suddenly I knew how much I had given up; I yearned to have it all back.

In 1966, Parsons College, in Fairfield, Iowa, was the final choice for many men who wanted to avoid the draft. In some funny way my mother also viewed it as a final choice for me. Barely two weeks after high school graduation I was sent off to college. I felt rejected by my mother's haste. I was not, however, rejected by the college men. The ratio there was seven men to one woman. I had so many dates it was confusing, fun and wild. For the first time in my life I felt incredibly important and loved.

On October 16, 1966, Nancy Brown, my socially-liberated freshman roommate, took me over to her current boyfriend's apartment to meet his roommate, Bill. It was Bill's birthday.

Over drinks I looked at Bill's handsome face and long body. He seemed intelligent and had a dry sense of humor.

"Let's celebrate your twentieth year on the planet," I said, as he took my hand and led me into his bedroom. We tore off our clothes. He slid into bed. The covers yawned open to embrace me. We coupled eagerly, and as he drifted off to sleep, I was sure I could feel my body change.

While home on Christmas break from school, after months of missed periods, I visited my family doctor. He told me in a quiet voice that I was pregnant. I went home and told my parents. Dad wept. I had never seen him cry before. Mom was surprisingly kind. I was numb.

Abortion was illegal in the United States. My parents considered sending me to France, where it was legal. Our family doctor suggested I go to The Willows, a home for unwed mothers in Kansas City, where they would arrange a secret adoption after the baby was born. I wanted more options, but there were none. My high-school boyfriend, Jack, had gone to my parents and offered to marry me, but they had decided that marriage for me at that point was not a good idea. They never told me about Jack's noble offer. I agreed to go to The Willows at the end of the semester. I returned to school, keeping the news of my pregnancy from most of my classmates.

"You don't have to worry; I'm taking care of everything," I assured Bill while biting my lip to keep it from trembling.

"How do I know this is my baby?" he confronted me coldly, glancing at the photo of his fiancée on the bureau.

"Well, think what you like," I countered, "I know it was you." I turned away with tears brimming.

Semester break came too soon. By the dark of a January night, my father and I left Parsons College behind. We traveled in silence through a violent storm to Kansas City. At dawn I waved good-bye to my father.

The Willows was a huge old house seated on the top of a hill with a giant wooden fence wrapped around it. We were not allowed to go out for a walk or to town without another pregnant woman or the social worker accompanying us. The fence kept life out and us in. The Willows was our prison and our sanctuary.

Every resident who arrived was white and wealthy enough to pay the expensive fees. My parents hid me away there and made me vow not to tell anyone I was pregnant, even my sisters, because it might ruin my father's professional reputation in our small town. Because of our families' need for secrecy, we each had to assume a fictitious surname to hide our identities.

I settled into a mundane routine, the endearing and compassionate Catholic priest, Father Matthew, being the most engaging part of my week. "Jack called yesterday and told me he's sleeping with my best friend," I confided to Father Matthew. "Jack was the one who took me to the doctor's office for my pregnancy test. As we drove off, I told him I was pregnant. He burst into tears and stalled the car. I got really irritated and yelled, 'It's not your baby, so why are you so upset?'" The priest patted my hand reassuringly. To calm my anger he pulled out a jumbo jar of sour dills from his valise, knowing full well how much I loved them.

The Kansas City summer was like a pressure cooker, hot and steamy. Every night we saw tornado warnings on TV and ran down to the cellar. This basement room was also our cafeteria. Some nights we would rush down before the warning and sneak peanut butter sandwiches.

A month after I arrived, a young woman named Kay appeared at The Willows. She was tall and lanky, with dark hair and a ready smile. We became intimate friends. She and I moved in together and began to entertain immediately. Other women and their roommates would come over and play cards, smoke cigarettes and gossip. Kay and I were due around the same time.

One hot July morning she had a baby girl. I was contemplating my approaching loneliness in the shower a few days later when a gush of liquid poured down my inner thigh.

"My water broke!" I yelped.

The labor room was empty as I walked in. "I think I could do this every weekend . . ." I chuckled as Kay smiled. Another contraction gathered around my belly and back. After dinner, Kay peeked into the room. The sweat was pouring off my face.

"What did I say about how easy this was? I feel like my back could break in two! How long did your labor last?" I implored. Kay held my hand and looked into my eyes. She stroked my face, and I relaxed.

Hours later, I was wheeled into the delivery room right next door. I heard the crunch of the needle going into my spine. I went numb as they raised my legs into the stirrups. My baby came gushing out.

"Oh, my God, it's alive!" I yelled jubilantly as the doctor placed a tiny boy on my deflating belly. My baby was quiet. I ached to breast-feed him. The nurse pulled him away. Our first separation. I begged her to bring him back, but she left the room with him in her arms.

As was the custom at The Willows, one week after the baby was born the mother could choose to hold her child for the first, and last, time.

"You can sit in the rocking chair. I will bring him out to you," the nurse said. I sank onto the hard surface. I opened my arms to this quiet, wide-eyed baby. I could hold him for one hour. I strained to see his face. I was blinded by the start of a migraine. I wanted to look deep into his eyes, take off all his clothes and examine every inch of his body, but the aura of the headache stopped me. I closed my eyes and invoked the Archangel Michael to protect him. We rocked until the nurse pulled him from my arms. As I walked away I fought the urge to look back.

Later that day I went to court. It was a red-hot July day in Kansas City.

"Raise your right hand, and repeat after me . . . I solemnly swear . . ." The words faded as I gazed at the judge. The lights hurt my eyes. I signed the document, realizing with each letter of my name I was giving up my son, Michael Flatley.

Twenty-six years later I cautiously inquired, "May I call you 'Michael'?"

"My name is Shawn Christian MacLean," he announced clearly.

I realized my son Michael was gone.

"I did choose the name Michael for my confirmation name. He was my special angel," he added.

It seemed so remarkable how well connected Shawn and I were. I remembered that when I was a child I used to gaze at the huge stained-glass window of Archangel Michael at St. John's Church. My grandparents had donated the window in memory of my Uncle Michael. I had named my son for this uncle, a medical doctor, who in his early thirties had killed himself in despair over his lengthy depression. That was in 1941, and his mental illness was later named manic depression. It seemed too soon to share all that with Shawn.

"Would you call me 'mother'?" I asked.

"I can't call you 'mother.' I have a mother already," he declared. "She's my real mother because she raised me."

"But I am your mother! No one can take that away from me," I said.

He was quiet, and I knew the struggle was over. He was totally grown, and all the roles in his childhood drama were clearly defined. I was an outsider and not able to be part of his family.

"Look, my parents are getting old, and they would love to meet you," I said.

"Sure, it sounds great. I'll work it into my schedule," Shawn said. I made all the arrangements, and in early September I flew home to Wisconsin. My parents looked even smaller than during my last visit. Together, the next day, we went to the airport to pick up Shawn.

A plane had just landed. "Point out which one he is when he gets off the plane!" Mom said eagerly. I leaned my face against the cool window. A young man in ripped jeans and a brown leather jacket, with books under his arm, stepped off the plane.

"Mom, there he is!" I pointed.

Dad stood a few feet away, his ever-increasing deafness isolating him. His attention was riveted to the airline gate. Mom and Dad beamed as they greeted Shawn. He looked tired and even more handsome than I remembered. He had gained some weight since I had last seen him. Mom and Shawn walked ahead of Dad and me. Dad's arm was under mine as he hobbled down the ramp, wincing from the pain in his knee.

When we arrived home Mom suggested I make the morning brunch. As I cracked the eggs into a bowl, Mom offered, "Shawn, what would you like to drink, wine or bourbon?"

I cringed as the three of them lifted their alcohol-filled glasses. I thought about the day I decided drinking was getting in my way. I'd wanted something more out of life than the blurred perception I got from that drug. It hurt to know they were going to slip into the fuzzy communication I so hated. Dad sat close to Shawn at the kitchen table. I was amazed to hear Dad begin to tell his life story. "After my mother and father attended the funeral of my uncle, they decided to leave me with my Grandmother Ellen." Dad's voice trembled and his eyes watered.

The next day I drove Shawn around my hometown and told him stories. I got lost on the highways, reminding me that the sleepy town I left eighteen years ago had grown to a large city.

While we were driving, I asked, "Have you ever had any mood swings?"

He looked at me keenly. "Well, maybe . . . What are you getting at?"

"My mother has a mental illness named manic depression, and it is genetically transmitted. I just wanted to mention it because if you experience extraordinary emotional highs and lows, please get help right away." He turned his face away toward the window. I sat, nervously waiting as he mulled it over.

"I did have a lot of ups and downs in college."

We looked at each other, and I felt such pain and helplessness. This was one of the exact reasons I had not wanted to give birth to any children.

"Well, if anything like that happens again at least now you'll know to get help," I repeated.

That night after dinner, Dad and Shawn stayed up drinking and watched a football game on television. They were yelling and having a good time. My father's deafness seemed to be limited to women's voices because when my son raised his voice, Dad could hear him a little. This party went on past midnight, and I had to get up the next morning for my plane at six. I got up and called to Shawn, "Hey, could you keep it down? I can't sleep through your noise." Peering through the bannister down to the first floor, I caught a glimpse of his face looking up at me, mouthing his reply.

"Maybe if you drank you could have fun."

I pulled away from the railing and retreated to my bed, feeling stung. His sarcasm resembled my mother's when she was having a breakdown. I felt uneasy with the similarity. The next morning he apologized.

My visit had ended. I waved good-bye to the three of them standing in the airport and boarded the plane home. My son had wooed my parents and won them over. I felt relieved to be getting away from Shawn and going home.

A week passed, and Shawn called me.

"I found my biological father," he announced proudly.

"Well, what did he say?" I asked.

"He was cautious. He seemed afraid. He said he wanted to talk to his lawyer before answering any of my questions. Sorry to say he seemed to have no personal charisma. I'm glad I found you first. I'm so glad I have you both, though," he shared.

"Please do me a favor. When you talk to Bill again, ask if he has Nancy Brown's phone number in Chicago? She was my freshman roommate and with a name like Brown in the city of Chicago . . . well, I got overwhelmed the last time I tried searching for her." I said.

Now that Shawn had found his biological parents, he suddenly insisted that we all have genetic blood tests. I felt angry that I had to prove something I knew was obviously true, but if this would give him total assurance that we all were genetically linked and appease his worries, I would do it.

Two weeks later I found myself in a hospital lab chatting with a nurse as she pressed my fingers onto an ink pad and then across a sheet of paper. These prints were for proof of my identity she told me. Next she got a Polaroid camera and took my picture for further documentation.

"I'm so nervous about the needle going into my arm," I said.

"You'll be very surprised at how little you'll feel; the needles are very well crafted, and the point is incredibly sharp," the nurse said.

"Thanks for telling me that. I delayed coming to the hospital for a week because I was scared. But my son was so adamant that he have scientific proof of our genetic identity, I relented. I gave him up twenty-six years ago through a secret adoption."

As I watched the Polaroid picture develop and the blood being drawn from my arm, she said, "Years ago I decided to become a single mom and got artificially inseminated. So far my child's not asking about the father."

"Well, I hope this test will satisfy my son's need to know for sure," I said, as she carefully placed the three tubes of blood into the Styrofoam package. I saw Bill's name on top of the form. According to Shawn, Bill was willing to pay the entire six-hundred-dollar fee. It amazed me that he was so generous in supporting Shawn's need for proof.

A month later, as Paul and I carried our groceries into the apartment, I noticed the message light blinking on my answering machine. I leaned over the counter and pressed the button.

"Hi, it's Shawn. I just got the test results, and I am going to have Bill talk to you."

"Did you hear that! The brat, he didn't even tell me what the results were. And he has the nerve to sound like he's reprimanding me. Have Bill talk to me! I haven't talked to him in more than twenty-six years. I'm not going to start now."

We played back the tape six times to make sure we truly heard a scolding tone. Paul finally nodded his head and said, "I think he is scolding you!"

I dialed Shawn's number and caught him at home.

"Shawn, this is Robyn. What's up?"

"Well it seems Bill's not the father," he said with an angry tone.

"Are you sure?" I stammered.

"The tests indicate he is not the father. So who is it? You said there were others, right?"

I stood there reeling from the shock. "I'm going to have to think about this; I still can't quite believe . . ."

"You have no right to withhold this from me!" he hissed.

"Look, I'm not trying to withhold anything, but I am shocked and will have to have time to think about this. Maybe I'm not the real mother either. Did you check the tests for us?"

"I'll give you a call next week with that information," he said. I hung up.

That night, after a long conversation with Paul, I went to bed searching my memory of that wild fall in Iowa. I had gone to many drinking parties and ended up in bed with a few men. What were their names? I had also slept with Jack right after summer school ended and at Thanksgiving, but these dates didn't add up as perfectly as the birthday celebration with Bill. I felt dizzy with confusion remembering my teenage wildness.

A few days went by before I heard from Shawn again. I was sitting in front of the television flicking the channels wildly when the phone rang.

"Hi, it's me," Shawn said. "Have you figured out who it might be?"

"No, I haven't," I answered. "Are we related?"

"Yes, we are related without a doubt. Well, what about your high school boyfriend; did he visit you that October at school?" he asked. "What was his name?"

"I'm not going to give you his name. What if I am wrong again and we go blundering into another person's life? I need to have more time to think. Plus he treated me badly."

"You owe this to me! You have no right to withhold that information from me . . ."

He went on for eight minutes, piling guilt upon righteous indignation and scorn. I held the phone away from my ear and waited. Finally he seemed to be slowing down, and I said, "You certainly are upset."

"One of us should hang up before someone says something they will regret," he stated, his voice quivering.

"I'm not going to hang up on you. Where would that get us? I need some time to figure out who it could have been. You realize I thought it was Bill for twenty-six years, and now I have to figure it all out again. Besides, I need to warn you about Jack if you end up contacting him. Please, give me some time."

"Well, that sounds good," he said calmly, clearly relieved.

We hung up, and I sat on the sofa peering into the night, wondering who the father could be and why I had only considered Bill all these years.

A few nights later the phone rang.

"Hi, stranger." The voice was light and lyrical. "It's Nancy Brown."

"Oh, God! I've wanted to hear your voice for so many years."

"Your son called me last Monday. He was really sweet, but I just couldn't talk to him then. I had just been diagnosed that day with pancreatic cancer."

"What are you going to do?" I gasped.

"Next Monday the doctors will operate, and if they can, they will take out my pancreas. Trust me, I will be fine. Your son called me again on Wednesday, and we talked longer. He asked about the men you were dating in the fall of 1966. I told him we were wild and I couldn't remember who I was sleeping with, much less who you were dating."

"I know. I tried to get him to see that it was a long time ago and we were pretty loose, but he's really determined to find his birth father. I'm surprised and annoyed, though, that he called you without my permission."

I called Shawn a few days later.

"I'm ready to give you Jack's full name and phone number. But first I want to tell you that although he was often funny, charming and quite bright, he could also be pretty strange at times. After you were born and I was back home, he and I went on a date. While we were sitting at a table in the bar, with our hands intertwined, he pressed his finger against my little finger's nail until the nail bent back, cracked and bled, all the while looking deeply into my eyes. I jumped up from the table and ran to the bathroom, crying. That's just one of the puzzling things he did to me. There are more, but I am especially worried that he may be mean to you. I feel very protective and couldn't bear him hurting you."

"I'm tough, and I can handle anything. Don't worry about me, I can be mean, too. If you really think this is okay, I would like to check it out," Shawn said.

Days later I called Nancy at the hospital. She sounded drugged and giggled as she told me that the cancer was not the size of a walnut but like a fist and was wrapped around the artery and following the nerves back to the vertebra. "They said they can shrink it with treatment," she said. "Trust me, I know they can do it."

What odd timing for our reunion. Nancy was facing death, and I was attempting to relive the precise moment of my son's conception.

I dialed Shawn the next day.

"Hi, have you heard anything? Did you contact Jack?"

"Well, uh, I . . ."

I could hear Shawn moving with the phone pressed to his ear and mouth.

"Bad time to catch you?"

"Well, I was sitting here with my baby brother and we were planning . . ."

"Does he know about me? Did you tell him?"

"No, he just wouldn't understand. He's not at all interested in finding his biological parents."

"Did you get a hold of Jack?" I asked.

"Oh, yeah. He took the blood test yesterday morning. At first he was reluctant. It cost two hundred dollars, but I paid it," Shawn said. "It'll take six weeks to process the test, and the results will arrive on my twenty-seventh birthday."

The tests arrived sooner. I was relieved when it turned out Jack was not the father. Shawn and I jointly agreed to call a halt to the search. I had no more leads, and I wasn't about to suggest another round of tests. But I still wondered if the tests results were wrong about Bill. Labs and lab technicians do make mistakes.

Nancy is now approaching the final few months of the medically-projected survival period for pancreatic cancer patients. In a recent phone conversation she sounded discouraged because her cancer has doubled in size. She said that she hoped some new chemotherapy would help.

It has been two years since Shawn's first call. Now we are back to silence. Ours is a different kind of silence, not pregnant with promise, but born of resolution. His need to connect with me has lessened with my inability to give him the necessary information about his birth father. All of the joy, exuberance and attraction that his first call stirred up in me has now dissipated. I know I am fortunate to have met my son, but I had hoped for more. He was not all the horrible things I imagined I might have to accept, but on the other hand he was not all the wonderful things I had imagined either. My greatest disappointment is that I am uncomfortable with him. What was once excitement is now tension.

Today I see Shawn merely as the young man he is, independent of me in every way except for my half of his genetic code. I imagine it must be like this for other mothers when they realize their son is not the person they had hoped he would be, but someone to be accepted for the individual he has become.

MARIAN MODELLE HOWARD

Shadows Burning

One daughter is back in my life now, but there's still one out there who refuses to have anything to do with me. Lisa is the one who speaks to me. She's married with a baby boy, Gabriel. I say I'm his grandmother —to anyone, that is, but my daughter. I don't want to hear her tell me I have no right to call myself his grandmother. Yet, I tell myself I don't have the right. When I mailed him a six-month birthday bear named Basil, I could have signed it "Grandma." Next time I will.

Not that she's making it easy for me to consider myself his grandmother. Why would she? She's angry and resentful. "Why couldn't you keep me?" she's asked over and over again. And though I've told her, my answer never seems to be good enough for her, or for me.

I hadn't seen or spoken to Lisa in twenty-four years when, in 1988, I sent her a letter. A year and a half later she wrote back.

"I'm a mother again!" I felt like shouting, telling everyone I knew and even those I didn't, that Lisa, my daughter, was back in my life.

But Lisa had written, "I don't want my parents to know I'm in touch with you. Please don't tell anyone. I'm afraid they'll find out before I tell them." So I told only my partner and my therapist. Imagine—my whole life had changed—my entire sense of myself was different—and all of this I had to keep a secret.

"Could you help me?" she wrote in that letter. "I need to know more about myself. What was I like as a baby? When did I begin walking, talking? What kind of pregnancy did you have? Did you want me? Did you try to abort me? Did you take care of yourself when you were pregnant with me? What happened? Why did you give me up?"

I dashed off a postcard to her, telling her I'd received her letter and would be answering it. It took me three weeks and many drafts before I mailed her a letter. I didn't want my guilt to chase her away. I continued being cautious throughout the spring, taking my time answering each of her letters. By the time my August vacation came, I was writing at top speed. I wrote a hundred pages that month, and I mailed her eighty of them, telling her everything I knew about her.

I answered each of her questions with as much detail as I could recall. Yes, she was planned for. No, I never wanted to abort her. Yes, I smoked while I was pregnant. I told her about the nurse who came into the labor room to show me a picture of Clark Gable's wife and their newborn child on the front page of the newspaper. Then they wheeled me off. Her delivery was easy.

"Was I a mistake?" Lisa asked in one of her letters.

No, Lisa, my marriage was the mistake, not you.

I married Joel when I was eighteen. He seemed so sure of himself, so in control of his life, that I thought he could take care of me. But soon into my marriage, I realized I was taking care of him. He had a big front but little substance. I had been fooled by an image.

When we were with our friends or families, he was always friendly, telling stories and jokes and in public he was warm to me, but at home he was unavailable, removed. I wanted to be touched, held, talked to. Joel wanted to watch television. If I complained, he told me he was tired, that he'd worked hard all day.

I was confused. I spoke to my married friends, women much older and experienced than myself. They reminded me that Joel worked hard for me and the girls, that he didn't run around or drink or gamble. This is the way marriage is, they said. Then they'd complain to me about their husbands.

I tried to make sense of what was happening to my life. I began to think that if my husband was one of the better ones, then something was terribly wrong with marriage as an institution. Or else something was wrong with me. I thought I might be exceptionally needy to want more love, caring and conversation than everyone else. I didn't know the answer, but I knew I was dissatisfied and distraught.

One morning as Joel was sitting on the side of the bed, I suddenly hit him. "Why'd you do that?" he wanted to know. I didn't have an answer for him. By this time I was so out of touch with my anger at him that I was as surprised as he was.

My children were the best part of my married life. Lisa was born in April

1961, when Rebecca was two and I was twenty-one. I hoped to have two more children. Though I was trying to make my life tolerable, things got much more difficult that winter. The girls were sick frequently, passing the flu back and forth between them. The only help Joel gave me was to watch them at night when I went out with friends. As long as the house was relatively clean, he didn't seem to care if I was home or not.

The idea of continuing in this marriage for the rest of my life, or at least until the girls were in college, made me despondent. I wasn't thinking about suicide, but I was wondering how I could continue living as I was. I went into therapy. About a year later, I said to a friend, "I think I want to leave Joel, but how do I know my life won't be worse without him?"

"Ask him for a trial separation," she said. "Don't say you want a divorce."

A few months later I told Joel I wanted to separate. As the words came out of my mouth, I knew I'd never go back to him.

I stayed in our apartment with our daughters, trying to survive on the few dollars Joel sent us and the money I earned from selling Avon and working for my father one or two days a week. Joel went to live with my parents, where he didn't pay rent and was served dinner every night by my mother.

I had believed a separation would make me feel alive again, but my new life as a single parent was much harder than I had expected. Pressed for money, I couldn't go out with friends, and the more I stayed home, the more isolated I became. I was drinking too much. I couldn't get out of bed in the morning. I had no patience with my children Rebecca was five, the age when she was going out more into the world. She needed my help, and I couldn't give it. I was baffled as I tried to cope with the school system she was entering. I began having blackouts. At some point I stopped drinking, but it didn't seem to matter. Most of the time I was in some place deep inside myself.

It was like being in a swamp. I wanted to die and came close to killing myself. I was saved by my friend Monica knocking on the bathroom door. "Why don't you let your mother take care of the girls?" she wanted to know.

Never, I said to myself, I'm afraid my father would molest them, like he did me.

That year, 1964, I told Monica that my father had sexually abused me for most of my life. We talked until three in the morning. Finally my secret was out. My worst fear, that I'd be told I was crazy, hadn't happened. Monica believed me.

"I know your father. I always knew he was perverted, but I never dreamed of this," she said.

No one did in the early 1960s. When I told my psychiatrist, he asked some questions, but didn't seem to do much with my responses. I'd bring it up again from time to time, until he said to me, "Are you still bothered by that?"

"If you loved me, you wouldn't have left me," Lisa wrote.

I loved my daughters, but I couldn't take care of them. I had nowhere to turn until their father let me know that he wanted them. I was sure he and his new wife would take better care of them than I could. So I said yes and thanked God for giving me and my kids a miracle.

Sundays became visiting days, traveling by subway and bus from Brooklyn to Hackensack, where Joel and Janice lived. It was too far to take the girls to my apartment, so we always had to be outside someplace. It was so different from when we lived together. I didn't know how to be with them. I felt like their babysitter, not their mother.

During those Sunday visits, Rebecca was sullen and disconnected and Lisa appeared confused. I had no idea what to do about their obvious distress. The last time I saw them, I took them to Central Park. Lisa wouldn't stop crying when it was time to go. I didn't know if it was me or the zoo she didn't want to leave. I couldn't bear her crying. I couldn't tolerate her pain, or mine.

Then Joel called me. "Rebecca's having a hard time adjusting. She gets very upset on the days she sees you. She cries before you come and says she doesn't want to go with you. A psychologist I spoke to thought it'd be better for her not to see you."

My psychiatrist agreed. "You'll be doing a wonderful and generous thing if you end your relationship with your daughters. You'll be giving them the chance to be normal—to have one mother and one father, like everyone else."

Now I know I should have said to Joel and both therapists, "To hell with all of you! These are my children. I love them. I want them in my life. They need me. I need them." But at that point, I didn't think I deserved them. So I agreed to stop seeing them and said nothing.

A few years later when Joel told me that his wife wanted to adopt the girls, I couldn't say no. She was raising them. She was taking Rebecca to school, meeting with her teacher, taking Lisa to the doctor, blowing her nose—she should be given the legal right to call herself their mother. I heard my psychiatrist's voice preaching the importance of "one mother, one father." I didn't feel I had the right to hold on to even the slightest connection to them. I didn't like it when I gave them up and I even felt some pride in my selflessness!

But don't tell me I "surrendered" them, which is what some people in the adoption world would say I did. Each time I hear the word used in that way I want to scream. "Never!—I never 'surrendered' my daughters. This wasn't a war, no shots were fired, no white flag was waved. My children were not some territory. I am their mother, and no one can take that away from me. I don't care what legal papers I did or did not sign. These are my children, who grew in my body. I gave birth to them. I am their mother."

Even today I try to deny the reality. Yes, of course I "surrendered" them. It was a war, after all; still is.

"Why did you disappear?" Lisa wanted to know.

My children were gone. I felt relief. But now I began using food the same way I'd used scotch—to numb my feelings. I stayed away from anything that related to children, anything that brought up my pain and guilt. I would read a book by the ocean until a mother arrived with her children. I'd try to ignore them and would succeed until a child began to cry. Then I'd get angry and leave the beach, muttering about crying children ruining my good mood.

Other times I felt free and happy. I began college and found out that I could think, a profound realization that changed the course of my life. Still, each time things got too good, I'd find a way to sabotage my joy. Sometimes I'd get so depressed, I'd feel like killing myself. I quit school. Worked in a college library. Came out as a lesbian. Fell in love. Went back to school. But no matter what I did—how many joints I smoked, how many pints of ice cream I ate, how many women or men I slept with—no matter how I tried to numb my pain over the loss of my children, I couldn't make it go away. I couldn't forget.

I imagine it was my pain that helped me become an understanding listener for my friends. When I was in my early thirties, they began to suggest that I become a college counselor or a therapist. It felt right. I needed to reach out to others. I wanted to help people heal. I went through graduate school and institute training and became a therapist. I worked on my own healing. My thoughts of killing myself went away. I couldn't do that to my clients. Eventually I didn't want to do that to myself.

"What do I do when I see you? Do I hug you?" Lisa asked me in our first telephone call.

Three days later I held out my arms to her as she stood in the doorway of my hotel room. She came into them as though she knew she belonged there. I almost couldn't catch my breath. After twenty-six years, my daughter, my child, was in my arms. We began talking and continued talking for the four days of my visit. I felt a new kind of love, or perhaps it was a feeling I'd known once but hadn't experienced in the years we'd been apart. I didn't want to leave her. We shared fantasies of living near each other. As I walked toward the airplane that would take me home, I thought my heart would break. I was leaving her again.

"I don't remember you" she said in a telephone call.

My story does nothing for Lisa's pain. Explanations don't soothe. I want to take her pain away, although I know I shouldn't and can't. Maybe she can't feel my love until I can fully give it. Sometimes I still don't understand who or what I am loving. When I think of her, she is a baby, a toddler. I picture her as she was then, and I can actually feel something in my heart softening. Who is this adult I am loving—this grown-up child who almost looks like me? How did she spend the twenty-six years she didn't know me? What is it that connects me to her—that allows me to feel so much love for her?

And what is it that stops me from simply showing her this love? About a month after our second visit together, she called up one evening, very upset. "Please come here and be with me," she said. When I said no, she insisted. I became stubborn. I had already taken off a week from work to be with her. I couldn't imagine taking off another week so soon. Maybe I could have gone for a weekend, but I didn't even think of it. Would I have responded to her differently if I had raised her all those years?

When I met Lisa's husband, I said, "Tell me if you can see ways that we're alike."

"All you have to do is look at your handwriting," he said. "It's almost identical."

She has the same color and texture of hair that I had at her age. She's tall and thin with lean bones. I'm short and round. But her cheeks are full like mine, a chipmunk. She's anorexic—"Under control," she says. I'm an overeater. So are her father and Janice, her adoptive mother.

If Janice is my daughters' mother, what does that make me?

People would ask, "Do you have any children?" An innocent question to most other women, a potential ice-breaker. But for me it was the killer question.

"Yes, but I don't see them," was the honest answer, one that I gave only if

I wanted to have a relationship with the questioner. When I thought I wouldn't see the person again or didn't care if I did or not, I'd say no. But I always felt shame, either because I was lying or because I had given up my kids.

"The one thing a mother doesn't do is give up her children." For years I believed that I was the only woman in the world who had ever given up her kids. It didn't matter that I knew better.

"Why did you write to Rebecca and not to me?" Lisa asked me.

When Rebecca was eighteen and no longer living at home with Joel and Janice, I sent her a letter. This time I was going to a different therapist. He wanted to know what I had felt over the years about losing my daughters. It was too hard. I'd worked so long on burying those feelings. I didn't want to feel the pain. I tried to avoid the feelings that were emerging, so I wrote to her impulsively.

I had hoped for a phone call or a letter in return saying, "Yes, I'd like to meet you," or at worst, a "Not yet," or no answer at all. Instead I got a lawyer's letter threatening to take me to court if I ever contacted either of my children again.

I realized Rebecca had taken my letter to her father. I didn't understand why he needed to have an attorney send me a letter. The message was clear— stay away. I felt hatred, anger and fear in their response. I didn't know if I'd ever have the courage to try again.

A few months later Joel wrote my mother and sister that he was forbidding Rebecca and Lisa to have any further contact with them. For the first time in my life, my mother apologized to me.

"I was wrong. All those years I acted like he was my son. I put him first. I should have put you first. You are my daughter."

It took me many years of therapy before I realized that both my parents consistently took care of their own needs instead of mine. How hard it has been to accept that each of them used me.

My therapist helped me make the connections between my father's sexually abusing me, my feeling dirty and unworthy and my not being able to take care of my daughters. What I couldn't say out loud until recently was that I was afraid I was like my father. After all I had his genes—my mother was always yelling at me that I was just like him. I never really understood why my father forced me to have sex with him. Maybe whatever made him that way was in me too.

Is it any wonder I was so willing and able to believe I was not good for my children, that my very presence was harmful to them? Finally, I put all of these feelings together and began to understand my life.

I still feel guilty. A part of me believes that having made a meaningful life for myself makes me a terrible person. It's as though I made a pact with the devil: "Give me your children, and you will have a successful life." I dismiss all the work I put in. I forget how hard this struggle for sanity has been for me. When I let myself know just how badly my parents damaged me, I know I had no choice. I could not raise my daughters. I could barely take care of myself. I would have destroyed the three of us. As long as I deny, in any way, the extent to which I was wounded, I will continue to feel guilty.

The other day, when I called Gabriel on his birthday, Lisa told me that I had called at the exact time she had given birth to him the year before. She also let me know that Gabriel was wearing the elephant shirt I'd just sent him for his birthday. And yes, I'd signed his birthday card "Grandma."

ADOPTIVE MOTHERS

JACQUELYN MITCHARD

Mother to Mother

Mother's Day is not the only time I think of her, but it's the only time I can't avoid it. She was going to have a child but couldn't keep it. I wanted a child desperately but couldn't have one. She was the mother at birth; I was the mother right after. It sounded simple, but it wasn't.

In the beginning, she was just a voice on the telephone from a hundred and fifty miles away. She was the one who answered my ad in an alternative newspaper —one of those notices you see that begins "Loving couple, in their thirties, unable to bear children. . . ." From that first moment, I liked everything about her, and that impression never wavered as we progressed from businesslike strangers exchanging resumes to intimates planning a tender offer of the heart.

For more than five months, we talked almost daily on the phone, each of us hungry to learn everything about the other. I tried to picture Amy, as I call her here, in my mind's eye, playing with the few details I knew—auburn hair, one hundred and twenty pounds, five-foot-four—like a child toying with different configurations of blocks. I imagined her smile, the clothes she wore, the bird feeder in her yard. It helped make her real. It helped me to trust her. And she seemed to need the same kind of details from me. "Describe the new slipcovers," she would say. "Tell me all about the dog."

Night after night, I would run in the door, drop my purse on the floor and call Amy. Sometimes she'd beat me to it; her voice would be waiting for me behind the blinking red light on the answering machine. "Hi, babe," she'd greet me. "Guess what?" The social worker had sent her forms, she'd say. The ultrasound showed a whopping, thriving fetus. At times we wouldn't even mention the legal plans and details that would attend my adoption of

71

the baby growing inside her.

Amy sounded like every girl I grew up with in Chicago—big-hearted, wise-cracking, mostly uneducated, but possessed of a fierce, intuitive set of smarts. Her slang, her very accent, comforted me.

Often I would hear her six-year-old son, from her former marriage, playing happily in the background. So she was a good mother. That was nice. Or was it? Could a good mother, who knew what it was to love a child, give up a baby? I couldn't see how.

The summer shadows deepened in the corners of the yard. The baby was two weeks late. Then on August 9, 1986, there was no answer when I called. Not the first time, not the second or fifth or tenth. There was no question about it: Amy had to be in the hospital. And I had to hear her voice telling me she hadn't changed her mind. Because that was always a possibility.

Amy was twenty-six, no panicky teenager. She was divorced, poor, but part of a big, proud, urban Irish family. Daily, she had told me, her mother pressured her to keep the baby. But Amy was steadfast. She could raise one alone. Not two. That's what she had said during the long months of her pregnancy. Would she still feel that way now?

Finally, just before 4:00 P.M., I pressed the redial on the phone and an unfamiliar woman's voice answered. "Who is this, please?" she asked sharply.

"I'm ah . . . I'm the lady from Wisconsin," I said. "Has Amy said anything about me?"

There was a pause before the voice said coolly, "I'm Amy's sister. You're the lady who was going to adopt the baby. Amy had the baby today: a little boy."

A boy. All my visions of pinafores and teeny tights melted away into an image of a big, sturdy, dark-haired son. But . . . maybe not.

"Did Amy intend . . . did she say she had changed her plans?"

"She said nothing about it," her sister replied, and then her voice softened. "I know this must be hard for you, but I just don't know."

And for two days, there was no knowing. I called again and spoke with Amy's mother, who said that her daughter was struggling with what was suddenly a very difficult decision, and would I do her the kindness of letting her make it without my influence? I promised that I would.

But on the evening of the third day, after I had clawed rows of welts along my forearms, I could wait no longer. I called the hospital, and they connected me with Amy's room.

I told her who I was. There was a long silence. Then, weak and sounding far away, she said, "Hi, babe."

She was terribly ill. She had suffered through an emergency Caesarean.

She had pneumonia. Her mother had talked the nuns into placing her in isolation; by rights, my phone call should not even have been put through. I made small noises of concern. But finally I had to ask.

"Amy, have you changed your mind? If you have, I'll hang up and wish you well and you'll never hear from me again. If you tell me to go ahead, I'll set things in motion."

She paused so long that I thought she had dropped the phone. Then she said, "Go ahead."

I made a big okay sign to my husband, who stood nearby, supporting himself on the kitchen counter. "But there's one thing," Amy said. "I want to see you."

We had never discussed this possibility. I didn't know how I felt about it. Once I put a face—a real face, not the smiling, benevolent visage I had concocted in my mind—to that familiar voice, would it haunt me for the rest of my life? Would I see it every time I looked at the child I already knew would be called Daniel Chamberlain—after his father, Dan, and his father's historical hero, Joshua Chamberlain, one of the heroes of the Battle of Gettysburg? But I pushed my doubts aside. There was nothing I wouldn't do to bring Daniel home.

Twenty hours later, my husband and I were in a crowded Chicago hospital, picking our way nervously down corridors to the maternity floor, expecting to be stopped at any moment. The nun gave me a measuring look when I asked for Amy. She was still in isolation, and no one but close family was allowed in the room when the baby was present. But as I learned later from a hospital social worker, the nun knew exactly who we were and decided to let God work it out.

She showed us to a cramped little room. Amy was sitting on the bed in a blue peignoir set that would have been right at home in an old Doris Day movie. Her hair was brick red; I knew right away that she had called it auburn to sound more sophisticated. She looked up. She was a pretty woman, with freckles and a generous mouth and the oddest color eyes—neither brown nor hazel but like a leaf just beginning to turn in the fall.

"Jack?" she said, using the nickname I had heard so often on the phone. My throat was too full for me to do anything but nod.

She stood up and came into my arms. We held each other silently. My husband put his arms around us both.

Then she turned to the Plexiglas bassinet that had been partially hidden behind her. She reached in and picked up a baby as big and bonny and rosy dark as I had imagined him. "Look, Danny," she said, "I told you Mommy and Daddy were coming."

My husband made a sound somewhere between a cough and a sob. Amy placed Danny in my arms.

As I nuzzled the baby, she crowed over him like any proud mother. "Isn't he beautiful?" she said. "See how big he is? See? He knows it's you. He smiled."

I was lost in him. The bonds radiated from him and locked me fast. What could I say? How could I compliment her on the fine son she had borne? Facing me was the mother who had suffered a massive physical assault to give him life. A woman who had turned her back on her family's offers of help and her obstetrician's referral to a wealthy North Shore couple who could give this boy things we never could. Amy had not broken our trust. I appreciated that then. I'm awestruck by it now.

Amy and I traded Danny back and forth. Then his new father held him. "Oh, thank you," Dan said over and over. "Thank you. Thank you." It sounded like a prayer.

After a long time, a nurse poked her head in the room. "No one but Mom is supposed to hold the baby," she said gently.

"But I—" I began, and stopped. Amy and I exchanged glances. I returned the baby to his bed. Amy covered him with a doll-size quilt. And then, straightening her shoulders, she began loading my arms with formula and diapers and little plastic containers of powder—all the free gifts that suppliers offer to maternity patients.

"I won't need these," she said firmly. "*You* will."

"I can't tell you . . ." I said.

Amy stopped me gracefully. "It's okay. I know."

It was over. There would be no more giggling on the telephone. No more trading of the details and secrets of our lives. Danny would be released to the social worker tomorrow; we would bring him home the same day. I would be a new mother.

Dan and I staggered to the elevator and through the lobby without a word. In the parking lot, he leaned against our van, his forearm over his eyes. I have heard him cry before and since, but not this way, not with such great gulps of love and pity. He could think of nothing, he finally said, but of Amy going home alone tomorrow and of some lines from a poem by Stephen Vincent Benet, in which the ghost of Abraham Lincoln's mother asks: "What's happened to Abe? . . . Did he grow tall? . . . Did he get on?"

"How can she bear it?" he said. I told him I didn't know.

We brought Danny home at noon the following day. I had promised Amy a last phone call to let her know we had arrived safely. While the relatives made much of our new addition, I slipped away and called her. She answered on the first ring.

"It's me," I said.

"I knew it would be."

"Are you okay?"

"I'm as well as I can be."

Just before we hung up, she said, "I want you to promise to raise him to be like us. To be tough. Don't let his daddy spoil him." And she added, "I'm glad he's a little boy."

"Why?" I asked.

"Because the world's too tough on little girls," she said.

Except for a single phone call that came a year later on Christmas Day, I have not heard from Amy again. Danny's grown into a bold and tender boy, uniquely at home with the world. He doesn't really look like the fading picture of Amy I keep in my mind—except for his eyes, which are the oddest color, like a leaf just beginning to turn in the fall.

One day, when he can understand, I'll tell my Danny the story of his birth. And if, when he's old enough, he wants to look up the woman who bore him, I will not protest—how could I ever fear Amy? I will ask only one thing: that I be allowed to go with him.

For I have things to tell her. I want her to know that, lo and behold, a couple of months ago the undreamed-of happened and I was able to give Danny a baby brother from my own body. I want to tell her that it was no different, that I love the child I bore no more than the one she placed in my arms. They are both angels of the outside chance.

And there's something else. See, I miss her. I want to know that the world hasn't been too tough on her.

When I do talk to Danny about Amy, I won't know exactly how to describe her. We weren't friends, precisely; nor were we family. It was as if we were strangers who met on a stranded bus and then went our own ways, but not without looking backward, each straining to see where the other was headed.

This much I will be able to tell Danny for certain: that he is who he is not only because he was raised by parents who searched for him and fought for him and adored him, but because of something else, too.

He comes of good stock.

DENISE SHERER JACOBSON

The Question of David

It was a rainy, winter, Bay Area Thursday. I'd spent a lazy morning—the benefit of being a self-employed writer—and had just gotten out of the shower when the telephone rang. I glanced at the clock: 11:52. At 12:30, someone was coming to discuss buying my player piano. With my jeans down around my knees, I flicked the switch of my motorized wheelchair, placed my palm on the joystick and whizzed across the bedroom. I reached the phone on the third ring. "Hello."

"Oh, hello," the female voice responded over static. "Is Neil Jacobson there?"

"He's at work."

"Ah, I must have his work number and home number mixed up," she explained in a slightly raspy, deep voice. I was about to hang up so she could call Neil at his office when she asked, "Are you Denise?"

"Yes."

She introduced herself as Colleen Somebody-or-other from St. Louis—a friend of a friend of mine. "Didn't Judy tell you I'd be calling?"

"No," I replied, swallowing my sarcastic "of course not." Judy always pulled stunts like this, and from previous experience, I had already put up my guard. In fact, my suspicion was that if Judy had told this woman to ask for Neil, chances were this was something I would need to be talked into.

"Well . . . er," Colleen paused as if gearing up for a dive into a cold pool. A moment later, she took the plunge. "There's a baby boy, almost five weeks old, up for adoption, and we just found out he may have cerebral palsy . . . Judy said that you and Neil might be interested."

A baby? With CP? How'd they know so early? I thought it took at least months before anyone noticed that a baby wasn't doing the things other babies did at the same age—turning over, crawling, responding to sounds—unless the baby's physical signs were so obvious. I had been almost a year old when doctors finally correctly diagnosed me. I listened.

Evan, as Colleen told me, was born with a torticolis ("he held his head to one side," she explained), and he had increased muscle tone (stiffer than that of other newborns). Since the adoption had been arranged before the baby was born, a CAT scan and an EEG were ordered just to "be safe." The tests showed slight swelling in the frontal lobe of the brain. No one could be sure what it meant, if it meant anything at all.

"The prospective parents are starting to have doubts about adopting him. They know nothing about cerebral palsy. We've been trying to educate them," Colleen said. "I work at an independent living center, and I've put them in touch with other parents who have kids with CP, but at this point, they're really scared . . . sooo, we're trying to line up another couple just in case."

She rattled on without a breath, telling me that there seemed to be no other outward signs or symptoms of any disability. Evan had no trouble breathing or swallowing.

"He's so alert and responsive. Has the sweetest smile," she interjected into the details before finally taking a quick breath. It still wasn't a long enough pause for me to get a word in—even if I could think of anything to say.

Next, she talked about the physical therapy program the baby was on—his neck and limbs were stretched three times a day.

I caught my grimace in the mirror and felt a lump of bile rise to my throat. I was appalled to think that this tortuous, old-fashioned method was still being used, on an infant, no less!

"It seems to have helped, too," Colleen added innocently. "His torticolis is hardly noticeable anymore."

Lucky his neck didn't break, I thought.

"But, Denise, this baby is so gorgeous!" she said, as if trying to convince me.

I glanced at the clock, wondering how to get rid of this woman.

"Oh, I almost forgot. I should tell you his birth date. It's December 19."

Was it the coldness of the room, or phantom fingers chilling my spine? December 19 was Neil's birthday!

"I'll talk to Neil," I found myself saying. "We'll call you back." I took her number.

It was 12:15. Neil would be at lunch. The best thing to do was not to think about the phone call. My pants and the piano came first. St. Louis was too far away, and besides, Neil had waited twenty-nine years to adopt, so two more hours wouldn't make much of a difference.

"A baby?" I mused at my face in the mirror after I hung up the phone.

"From St. Louis?" it wrinkled back.

"Ridiculous!" I shook my head and returned to pulling up my jeans.

The first time Neil and I had discussed adoption was on our initial date. It wasn't a typical "getting-to-know-you" conversation. Instead of warming up with Woody Allen films and Bruce Springsteen's latest album, I listened to Neil's experiences of childhood—growing up with parents who were Holocaust survivors, who spoke little English and who were frightened by a medical profession that had a very pessimistic view of children with cerebral palsy.

"When I was five, a doctor recommended my parents put me in an institution," he explained as he slouched casually in his wheelchair. "So, I went with my father to see what it was like." He shook his head. "There were kids there sitting on the cold floor—half-naked—just rocking back and forth. It was horrible. My father actually got sick to his stomach. Afterward, my parents were so scared I might be taken away, my mom took all three of us kids to live with relatives in Florida for a year."

I felt a knot in my stomach. We all had our "war stories," but this seemed so incredible! To think that this man sitting across the restaurant table from me, a man who was now an esteemed computer scientist in the corporate world, had nearly ended up in a state institution, enraged me. Yet, he spoke about it so matter-of-factly.

"Doesn't it make you angry?"

"Naw," he said simply. "What would be the point? It happened a long time ago."

The waiter removed our barely touched chicken kiev. He came back momentarily with two cups of black coffee. We each asked him for a straw and to pour the cream. When we were alone again, I watched Neil take the glass lid off of the sugar bowl and, with careful precision, grasp an unwrapped cube of sugar between the tips of his thumb and middle finger and plop it into the coffee. He did this seven times. I tried not to cringe. "Now you know why we came here," he grinned, as his sparkling brownish-green eyes indicated the half-empty bowl. "Otherwise, people groan when they put the sugar in for me. That's the trouble with Berkeley—everyone's so healthy . . .

"Anyhow," Neil said after taking a sip, "I've wanted to adopt a disabled child ever since."

I blinked at him. I had just gotten over the sugar plopping. "Why?"

"There are so many kids out there living in institutions, needing homes.

And a disabled child needs a good home even more."

His enthusiasm intimidated me. I admired people who could be so selfless, but I'm not Mother Theresa. I knew my own limits. "It would be hard raising a disabled kid. Aren't you afraid it would be like reliving the same stuff you grew up with?"

"But I survived," he answered, "and that's what I can give to a child—I've given it a lot of thought."

"At least twenty-four years," I teased.

"Yeah," he nodded with a smile. "And I'm realistic. I know I wouldn't be able to handle a kid who's very physically disabled. And I wouldn't be good with one who was mentally retarded—I'm too impatient. Yeah, I've got to be practical."

Practical? I didn't know about that! Neil and I had known each other for years, though not well. Our paths had crossed when we were kids in New York—at camps and recreation centers. And now, living in the Bay Area, we had mutual friends. We had bumped into each other from time to time, but I had never thought about dating him and I was pretty sure he felt the same way about dating me; I always saw him with non-disabled women. It had been only a few weeks ago, at Judy's potluck Rosh Hashonah dinner, that I had realized Neil was quite an attractive man.

Before then, I had seen him as just a stereotype—someone with cerebral palsy: uncoordinated body movements, impaired speech and motorized wheelchair—a mirror image of myself, with a beard. And in the past, whenever I'd looked in the mirror, all my features—my smooth oval face, my blue eyes and auburn hair, my body with its adequate curves—had blurred into my cerebral palsy. It had taken a lot of years of work and pain before I could believe that my CP was a part of me, instead of believing I was part of it. Now that I had waded through some of the quicksand of my own prejudices, Neil was there . . . but adopting a disabled child?

"I've never given much thought to adoption," I said, tightly clasping my hands under the table before admitting, "I've always wanted to have a baby."

"So would I!" Neil's whole face brightened with a grin. "It would be such a kick!"

That conversation was the first of many we had on having kids, before and after we got married—while I kept track of my menstrual cycle. Neil believed more in fate than science when it came to conception and was able to add levity to my biological approach when it came to trying. Yet, every month, at the first sign of my menstrual blood, I felt a pang of disappointment and, eventually, hopelessness. At the end of three years when we finally resorted to sperm counts, a dye X-ray of my uterus and four months of artificial insemination so that Neil's sperm had a shorter swim to my egg, I decided maybe Neil did have the better idea.

Adopting an older child—say, three or four years old—did make sense: No hassling with bottles and diapers, and, with a child that age, we would be more certain of what the disability was like. So, six months ago, I had phoned the local chapter of Aid to Adoption of Special Kids (AASK), an agency working with "hard to place" children.

We went through endless interviews, reference checks, finger prints and a doctor's exam. We were still waiting for all the paperwork to clear before final approval from AASK. Then there would be even more waiting while the agency attempted to match us with a child, taking into account that we were both disabled.

"It could take anywhere from three months to a year," the child placement worker warned with a patronizing smile, "because of your 'special' circumstances. And once we find a child, we may have to convince his or her social worker that you'll be good parents."

The other agency staff were much more encouraging, but I kept hearing those words over and over again. They deepened my fears. I knew that even after we contended with the prejudices of the child's social worker, we would have to deal with that child's initial reaction to having disabled parents.

A baby would be so much simpler. A baby would have no preconceived ideas of what parents should be like . . . yet, babies were in such demand to be adopted by non-disabled couples. For Neil and me, trying to adopt a baby seemed as silly and futile as a dog chasing its own tail.

It was a little after 2 P.M. when I dialed Neil's office.

"Hiya."

"Um . . ." Clenching the phone to my ear, I stumbled through the purpose of my call. "Neil . . . I got a call a couple of hours ago. A woman in St. Louis—a friend of Judy's . . . there's a five-week-old baby up for adoption. He might have CP, and Colleen, the woman—whoever the hell she is—said the couple set to take him is freaked out. So now they're looking for a backup and your friend, Judy, gave our name . . . goddammit, why couldn't she have warned us? And this woman talked ten thousand words a minute." My voice cracked. "I didn't know what to ask . . . I said we'd call her back, but *you* do it, Neil. You call her back. Judy told her to ask for you, anyway."

"Denise, calm down," Neil said, when I paused for a swallow. "I can't tell if you're happy or upset."

"I'm pissed," I replied, feeling welling tears. Couldn't he hear it in my voice?

"Why?"

A tear rolled down my cheek. I struggled to hold back the rest so I could answer. "Because Judy should have asked us first."

"But she knows we're already in the process," Neil calmly responded.

"How could some stranger just call and offer us a baby?" I ranted on, ignoring his logic. "From what she told me, he doesn't even sound very disabled. I bet once the other couple calms down they'll probably keep him."

How could I have even tried to tell him that it felt as if someone were playing a practical joke on me. After I had "reasoned" myself out of wanting a baby, there it was dangling before me.

"Why don't I give the woman a call?" Neil suggested, responding pragmatically, as usual, to my emotional outbursts.

I sniffed and read off the number I had scribbled.

"By the way, Neil," I said in a calmer, almost shy, voice, "the baby was born on your birthday."

Neil called me back twenty minutes later without any more details, but from the high-pitched squeals that escaped his larynx, I knew my logical systems analyst husband had been overtaken by passion.

I still didn't think the idea was worth getting excited about. Determined not to give it another thought the rest of the afternoon, I threw on my clumsy plastic rain poncho, grabbed the borrowed English mystery from the bookcase and tore down the ramp. Maybe the rain and a mocha would melt away the knot in the pit of my stomach.

When Neil came home that night, his eyes sparkled and he wore a grin at least five inches wide.

"Let's eat first!" I stated firmly, finding it difficult, as usual, not to be infected by his enthusiasm. Besides, I didn't want to talk about it until our airy-fairy housekeeper, Chavallah, padded her way out of the house and into the night.

As soon as she was off, Neil squealed.

"I thought you didn't want to adopt a *baby*," I began. "You always said you wouldn't know what to do with it. You'd be afraid to touch it."

"But I'd figure it out." He gave me a cocky smile. "Remember the shirt?"

I bit back the smile that came to my lips. How could I forget the first obstacle to our physical relationship: Neil couldn't sleep over on weeknights because neither of us could fasten the top button of his shirt in the morning (and he had to wear a tie). At his place, one of Neil's roommates woke up at the crack of dawn to do it for him, but at mine, there were just the two of us and my cat. We were not about to let one button cramp our sex life, though. First, I tried my buttonhook, but, not having such a steady hand, aiming one so close to Neil's throat had lethal potential. Velcro, another possibility, became "linty" in the washing machine. Then one evening Neil appeared at my door, beaming. His fingers pushed aside his tie to show me a zipper sewn underneath a flap of fake buttons.

"Yeah," I said remembering, "but that's different."

"No, it isn't," he responded. "You're the one who insisted that if we really wanted a baby, we could do it."

"I know, I know," I grudgingly admitted, but suddenly, I wasn't so confident. What if I was so nervous around the baby that my movements would get out of control and I'd sock the poor kid in the jaw when I changed his diaper?

"We don't know much about his disability," I pointed out.

"Colleen's sending us the medical report."

"It's a private adoption," I reminded. "Can we afford it?"

He stroked his chestnut beard. "Can we afford not to?"

"Neil!" Sometimes he just infuriated me. I decided to change my approach. "Do you really think some woman from a Christian adoption agency is going to give a baby to a couple of Jewish cripples?"

"We'll find out, won't we?"

Never a straight answer. I plowed on. "Well, you know Colleen said the baby might be mentally retarded. And *you're* the one who didn't want a retarded child. And what if his disability is more involved than we can physically handle?"

"All I know is, there's a baby out there who needs a home."

I groaned: Were we going to go through this for every baby who needed a home?

"Neil, I just didn't think it would be this soon. We haven't even sold the piano. There's no room for a crib . . ."

"Look, let's just see what happens," Neil finally suggested.

I sprawled out on the couch to watch a couple of mindless comedies while Neil did his "paperwork." Laughter loosened some of the tension in my neck and shoulders, and by the time we got ready for bed, my mood had lightened.

"Do we have to name him Evan?" Neil asked while he kicked off his shoes. (He stammered with names that began with vowels.)

"I don't know," I responded with a shiver after taking off my turtleneck, "but we always said if we had a baby we'd name it after your father, Jacob." (According to Jewish tradition, a baby is named after a deceased relative to carry on that person's memory.)

"But I don't like pronouncing 'J's,' either."

"Well, my nephew Larry's already named after my mother, so it would be nice to name the baby for someone else." I thought a few moments while I slipped my arms out of my bra straps, twisted the bra around and pinched open the hooks. After I wormed on my warm flannel nightgown, I spoke again. "Hey, my great aunt Dinah never had any kids. She adored my sister and me."

"You want to name him Dinah?" Neil retorted playfully. I saw his raised eyebrow in the mirror.

"No," I laughed. "But all we have to do is find a name with 'D.' Maybe David. As long as the Hebrew meaning's the same."

"David," Neil repeated without a stammer or a stutter. He grinned. "David. I like it."

"Me, too." I smiled briefly. Who knows, this may work out . . . "Who's going to call the agency?"

Making telephone calls to strangers was never on our "most fun things to do" list. Neil and I spoke clearly enough face-to-face, and our friends had no difficulty understanding our slurred, 33-1/3 speech over the phone. We even gave lectures on disability issues at colleges and medical schools. But when it came to calling places like Sears or the local gas company, we'd recruit a friend instead of chancing that we'd get an impatient operator or reception-ist—or worse, be hung up on. And now we had to call this woman and ask for a baby!

To my surprise and relief, Neil volunteered. "But Colleen said that I shouldn't contact the agency until the other couple decides not to adopt David."

I clamped my mouth shut. He was already calling this baby "David."

A few days later, a copy of the medical report on "Baby Boy K" arrived, along with some Polaroids. I grabbed the report while Neil looked at the pictures. I frowned; he squealed.

"It doesn't say any more than we already know, except it uses bigger words. Gives him a 50-50 chance of having cerebral palsy and/or mental retardation."

"Look at the pictures," Neil squawked, shoving the Polaroids in front of me. Propped up on cushions, the red-headed, blue-eyed infant, with his head upright, smiled a toothless smile.

"He's cute, I guess." I shrugged, disappointed that I didn't feel the same excitement. "But Neil . . . his head looks big. I think the report mentioned hydracephalus."

Neil rolled his eyes. "Denise!"

I reread the report three times and couldn't find it. I smiled sheepishly, "Well . . . maybe I am being too critical."

Why was I being so hard? I felt so confused. Was I ready for a baby . . . a disabled baby? Would I have to relive my own experience of childhood—the grueling therapy, the "special education," the loneliness of a child not being accepted by the non-disabled world? And what if he wasn't disabled? Who would rescue him when he climbed the plum tree outside the kitchen window? And when he got older, would he be embarrassed to bring friends home? How would I handle that? Why should I have to?

Neil had already made up his mind. It was easy for him. He spent nearly twelve hours a day at the office. He wouldn't have to deal with the details of dependence on au pairs and housekeepers with strong or peculiar personalities, annoying habits, stupidity. I was a writer. I liked my privacy; I had struggled all of my life to be physically independent, and succeeded. After spending a good portion of my thirty-six years in self-absorption, could I suddenly become a devoted mother of an adopted child?

A week later, we got the news—the other couple had backed out.

We decided to put off springing our decision on our relatives, particularly Neil's mother, who hadn't been too pleased about Neil's marrying me—because I had CP. We did tell our friends, who offered support and well-intentioned advice: "Get a lawyer," some told us. "His disability looks mild," another said. "Be sure to contact state disability services; you'll probably be eligible for financial assistance."

". . . And don't worry, Denise," my friend who had just become a mother tried reassuring, "when you see him, you'll know."

Sure, I humphed to myself, when have I ever let my instinct interfere with logic and guilt?

Even time wasn't on my side. Two weeks later Neil gleefully informed me that he had spoken to the social worker at the adoption center and if everything went smoothly, the baby could be in our home in four to six weeks!

"We haven't even sold the piano. We have nowhere to put your desk or the computer," I ranted. "And where are we going to find an au pair? It's not fair! Most people have nine months to get ready." I shook my head. "Neil, where are we going to get a crib? And what about baby clothes . . . diapers . . . bottles?"

"Details, details, details," was my husband's classic reply.

Hunched over the table and in a state of frazzled fatigue, I managed to shoot him a sharp look before glancing at my wristwatch. Seven o'clock. Time for me to call the baby's foster mother, Kate—as I had dutifully done every other evening for the last two weeks—to check on the baby.

Kate, I had learned, was the one who had instigated this unusual production of finding another home for this baby.

"The baby's doing fine," Kate warmly assured me after our first 'hellos.' Her voice was strong, with just a trace of an ancestral Irish brogue. I pictured her a large, rounded earth mother, with long reddish brown hair and wearing Birkenstocks, babies and toddlers crawling over her feet and clinging to her peasant skirt.

Each time we talked she always sounded so comforting, as if she were an old friend. "You know, he's so alert. He smiles at you. Why, he was smiling when he was two weeks old. I told everybody, and they said it was gas. But I've been taking care of babies long enough to know the difference—it definitely was a smile."

After our conversation, tears stung my eyes. He was so real, this negotiation, this baby. This baby I was so afraid of wanting. He did things babies did. He was soft and round, and he smiled. Suddenly, I remembered the story my mother had told me about the doctors who diagnosed me as mentally retarded, years before EEGs and CAT scans. My mother decided they were crazy. She'd tell me: "They didn't see the twinkle in your eyes."

"Neil, I need to go to St. Louis," I stated after swallowing the lump in my throat.

"Of course," he agreed. "One of us should go and check it out."

I gave him a sad smile; we were on such different wave-lengths.

Neil drove me to the airport, one week later, as the stars faded into the grey daylight. Unfortunately, I hadn't been able to get a front seat in coach. I ended up in an aisle seat in the thirty-second row—a long way back and an even longer way out—without my chair.

When the plane landed in St. Louis three hours later I unbuckled my seat belt and waited. The other passengers had to deplane first—those not going to New York, that is—before someone could assist me. As usual, it was taking forever, and I just hoped that the plane wouldn't take off for its final destination with me still on board. Yet, somehow I didn't think Colleen, who was meeting me, would let them.

I swallowed, trying to pop my ears, and breathed in the thin, cold stale airplane air hissing out of the small metal cones above my head. With cold, clammy hands, I stuffed my *Games Magazine* and Cynthia Ozick's anthology into my backpack and placed it on the seat beside me. Then I put on my jacket; I wanted to be ready when the narrow aisle-chair (a dolly-like conveyence) and the always impatient ground crew came to transport me to my wheelchair.

Twenty minutes later, I was still there, my stomach rumbling, my fingers tugging at the neckline of my sweater. I squirmed under the little light bulb staring down at me from between the air cones, while my hand absently rummaged through my open-mouthed backpack. I felt the sharp edges of the magazine and then a furry snout. I snatched the softness.

I held up the brown teddy bear with both hands and inspected its friendly face. I had bought it just yesterday, with reservation. I felt an empty, gnawing ache inside. Did I come here to make sure I did or didn't want this baby?

Finally, the aisle-chair appeared! I stuffed the teddy bear down into my pack as the men parked the chair alongside my seat and prepared to lift. I didn't bother trying to explain to them that I could transfer myself from the seat to the chair; I sensed they'd rather lift than communicate.

"My bag," were the only words I uttered to the man nervously buckling the criss-crossed straps over my chest.

He glanced to the seat where I'd been sitting and called over my head. "Better get her bag. She's worried about it . . ." I watched my backpack slung from the man behind to the man in front. "Ready?" he asked his peer in the rear as he stepped aside, without a word to me.

I was tilted back and wheeled through the cabin—their cargo. I detached myself, first looking to my left, through rows of windows framing the blue winter's sky, and then to my right at the passengers settling in for the last leg of the flight.

"'Bye now." The friendly gray-haired man, who had smiled at me on my way in, called to me on my way out. *He must be from the Bay Area!*

We were in the first cabin when I was surprised by a strong, slightly broguish voice. "Denise?"

I turned my head. I saw just enough of the small, neat, fiftyish-looking woman to realize she wasn't the Kate I had pictured. She stood in front of me, but my eyes instantly latched onto the bundle she held. He was just at my eye level.

"Oh, my God!" I gasped.

"Here's your son," she offered with outstretched arms.

His small, solid body sat snugly in my lap. My arm cradled him. I felt my eyes blazing as I stared increduously at him. He tilted his fuzzy reddish-golden head back. Red "stork bites" peppered his forehead and eyelids, but his cheeks were round, as smooth and white as a spring lily. He smiled at me. His blue eyes whispered to mine: *"It's about time you got here."*

"You were born so far away," I blinked.

"I want to go home," he stared back.

In our silent dialogue, his eyes held mine in a sharp, steady gaze. A shining gaze that, as it held my eyes, bored like a steel lance into my heart, piercing my core with a deep, painful joy I had never known before—a feeling without word or thought. Tears streamed down my cheeks.

"My baby, my baby," I cried over and over.

My lips brushed his hair while a buzz of voices murmured above us I didn't look up. I just hugged my precious David.

LOUISE ERDRICH

The Broken Cord

The snow fell deeply today, February fourth, two days before Michael and I are to leave for our first romantic trip together, ten days before Saint Valentine's holiday, fifteen days after Adam's twentieth birthday. This is no special day, it marks no breakthrough in Adam's life or in mine, it is a day held in suspension by the depth of snow, the silence, school closing, our seclusion in the country along a steep gravel road which no cars will dare use until the town plow goes through.

It is just a day when Adam had a seizure. His grandmother called out to me and said that she could see, from out the window, Adam lying in the snow, having a seizure. He had fallen while shoveling the mailbox clear. Michael was at the door too but I got out first because I had on sneakers. Jumping into the snow I felt a moment of obscure gratitude to Michael for letting me go to Adam's rescue. Though unacknowledged between us, these are the times when it is easy to be a parent to Adam. His seizures are increasingly grand mal now. And yet, unless he hurts himself in the fall there is nothing to do but be a comforting presence, make sure he's turned on his side, breathing. I ran to Adam and I held him, spoke his name, told him I was there, used my most soothing tone. When he came back to consciousness I rose, propped him against me, and we stood to shake out his sleeves and the neck of his jacket.

A lone snowmobiler passed, circled to make sure we were all right. I suppose we made a picture that could cause mild concern. We stood, propped

---

Editor's note: This essay is a slightly adapted version of the foreword to *The Broken Cord: A Family's Ongoing Struggle with Fetal Alcohol Syndrome* by Michael Dorris, HarperCollins Publishers, Inc., 1989.

together, hugging and breathing hard. Adam is taller than me, and usually much stronger. I held him around the waist with both arms and looked past his shoulder. The snow was still coming, drifting through the deep-branched pines. All around us there was such purity, a wet and electric silence. The air was warm and the snow already melting in my shoes.

It is easy to give the absolute dramatic love that a definite physical problem requires, easy to stagger back, slipping, to take off Adam's boots and make sure he gets the right amount of medicine into his system.

It is easy to be the occasional, ministering angel. But it is not easy to live day in and day out with a child disabled by Fetal Alcohol Syndrome. This set of preventable birth defects is manifested in a variety of ways, but caused solely by alcohol in an unborn baby's developing body and brain. The U.S. Surgeon General's report for 1988 cautioned on the hazards of drinking while pregnant, and many doctors now say that since no level of alcohol has been established as safe for the fetus, the best policy to follow for nine months, longer if a mother nurses, is complete abstinence. Every woman reacts differently to alcohol, depending on age, diet, and metabolism. However, drinking at the wrong time of development can cause facial and bodily abnormalities, as well as lower intelligence, and may also impair certain types of judgment, or alter behavior. Adam suffers all the symptoms that I've mentioned, to some degree. It's a lot of fate to play with for the sake of a moment's relaxation.

I never intended to be the mother of a child with problems. Who does? But when, after a year of marriage to his father I legally adopted Adam, the same child Michael had adopted, years before, as a single parent—it simply happened. As in so many extended families with Native backgrounds, adoption was common in my own. My Ojibwa grandmother and grandfather lovingly raised the children around them who needed raising, blood-related or not. And my own father and his brother had lost their mother early on and lived so closely with their stepmother that I hadn't known, until I was nearly twenty years old, that we hadn't a biological connection. That hardly mattered. Loving Adam came completely naturally—I've never questioned that for a moment. Living with Adam is a difficult thing. Day to day, it is a balancing trick, a set of desperate trade-offs, intensely frustrating and also lighted by deep moments of sheer grace. His goodness is astounding, as is his inability to hold a grudge, his utterly unconfused love.

As for my occupation, our relationship touches upon it only in the most peripheral ways; this is the first time I've ever written about him. I've never disguised him as a fictional character or consciously drawn our experience together. It is, in fact, painful for a writer of fiction to write about actual events in one's personal life. Michael, an anthropologist and novelist, struggled with writing about Adam for six years. The work was a journey from the world of professional objectivity to a confusing realm where the boundaries could no longer be so easily drawn. It was wrenching for Michael to relive this story, but in the end, I think he felt compelled to do so after realizing the scope of the problem, after receiving so many sad and generous stories from other people, and in the end out of that most frail of human motives—hope. If one story of FAS could be made accessible and real it might just stop someone, somewhere, from producing another alcohol stunted child.

Adam sees Michael and me primarily in the roles to which we've assigned ourselves around the house. Michael is the laundryman, I am the cook. And beyond that, most importantly, we are the people who respond to him. In that way, though an adult, he is at the stage of a very young child who sees the world only as an extension of his or her will. Adam is the world, at least his version of it, and he knows us only as who we are when we enter his purview.

Because of this, there are ways Adam knows us better than we know ourselves, though it would be difficult for him to describe this knowledge. He knows our limits, and I, at least, hide my limits from myself, especially when I go beyond them, especially when it comes to anger. Sometimes it seems to me that from the first, in living with Adam, anger has been inextricable from love, and I've been as helpless before the one as before the other.

We were married, Michael, his three children and I, on a slightly overcast October day in 1981. Adam was thirteen, and because he had not yet gone through puberty he was small, about the size of a ten year old. He was not, and is not, an immediately charming person, but he is generous, invariably kind-hearted, and therefore lovable. He had then, and still possesses, the gift—which is also a curse, given the realities of the world—of absolute, serene trust. He took our ceremony, in which we exchanged vows, literally. At the end of it we were pronounced husband, wife, and family by the same friend, a local judge, who would later formally petition for me to become his adoptive mother. As Judge Daschbach pronounced the magic words, Adam turned to me with delight and said, "Mom!", not Louise. Now it was official. I melted. That trust was not to change a whit, until I changed it.

Ten months pass. We're at the dinner table. I've eaten, so have our other children. It's a good dinner, one of their favorites. Michael's gone. Adam eats a bite then puts down his fork and sits before his plate. When I ask him to finish, he says, "but Mom, I don't like this food."

"Yes, you do." I tell him. I'm used to a test or two from Adam when Michael is away, and these challenges are wearying, sometimes even maddening. But Adam has to know that I have the same rules as his father. He has to know, over and over and over. And Adam *does* like the food. I made it because he gobbled it down the week before and said he liked it, and I was happy.

"You have to eat it or else you'll have a seizure in the morning," I tell him. This has proved to be true time and again. I am reasonable, firm, even patient at first, although I've said the same thing many times before. This is normal, Adam's way, just a test. I tell him again to finish.

"I don't like this food," he says again.

"Adam," I say, "you have to eat or you'll have a seizure."

He stares at me. Nothing.

Our younger children take their empty dishes to the sink. I wash them. Adam sits. They go upstairs to play, and Adam sits. I check his forehead, think perhaps he's ill, but he is cool, and rather pleased with himself. He has now turned fourteen years old. But he still doesn't understand that, in addition to his medication, he must absorb so many calories every day, otherwise he'll suffer an attack. The electricity in his brain will lash out, the impulses scattered and random.

"Eat up, I'm not kidding."

"I did," he says, the plate still full before him.

I simply point.

"I don't like this food," he says to me again.

I walk back to the cupboard. I slap a peanut butter sandwich together. He likes those. Maybe a concession on my part will satisfy him, maybe he'll eat, but when I put it on his plate he just looks at it.

I go into the next room. It is eight o'clock and I am in the middle of a book by Bruce Chatwin. There is more to life . . . but I'm responsible. I have to make him see that he's not just driving me crazy, he's hurting himself. So eventually I return to the kitchen.

"Eat the sandwich . . ."

"I did." The sandwich is untouched.

"Eat the dinner . . ."

"I don't like this food."

"Okay then. Eat half."

He won't. He sits there. In his eyes there is an expression of stubborn triumph that boils me with the suddenness of frustration, dammed and suppressed, surfacing all at once.

"EAT!"

I yell at him. Histrionics, stamping feet, loud voices, usually impress him with the serious nature of our feelings much more than the use of reason. But not this time. There is no ordering, begging or pleading that will make him eat, even for his own good. And he is thin, so thin. His face is gaunt, his ribs arch out of his sternum, his knees are big, bony, and his calves and thighs straight as sticks. I don't want him to fall, to seize, to hurt himself.

"Please . . . for me. Just do it."

He looks at me calmly.

"Just for me, okay?"

"I don't like this food."

The lid blows off. Nothing is left. If I can't help him to survive in the simplest way, how can I be his mother?

"Don't eat then. And don't call me Mom!"

Then I walk away, shaken. I leave him sitting and he does not eat, and the next morning he does have a seizure. He falls next to the aquarium, manages to grasp the table, and as his head bobs and his mouth twists, I hold him, wait it out. It's still two days before Michael will arrive home and I don't believe I can handle it and I don't know how Michael has, but that is only a momentary surge of panic. Adam finally rights himself. He changes his pants. He goes on with his day. He does not connect the seizure with the lack of food, he won't. But he does connect my words, I begin to notice. He does remember From that night on he starts calling me Louise, and I don't care. I'm glad of it at first, and think it will blow over when we forgive and grow close again After all, he forgets most things.

But of all I've told Adam, all the words of love, all the encouragements, the orders that I gave, assurances, explanations and instructions, the only one he remembers with perfect, fixed comprehension, even when I try to contradict it, even after months, is "don't call me Mom."

Adam calls me Mother, or Mom now, but it took years of patience, of back-sliding and of self-control, it took Adam's father explaining and me explaining and rewarding with hugs when he made me feel good, to get back to mother and son again. It took a long trip out west, just the two of us. It took a summer of side by side work. We planted thirty-five trees and one whole garden and a flower bed. We thinned the strawberries, pruned the lilacs and forsythia. We played Tic-tac-toe, then Sorry. We lived together. And I gave up making him eat, or distanced myself enough to put the medicine in his hand and walk away, and realize I can't protect him.

That's why I say it takes a certain fiber to live and work with a person obsti-nate to the core, yet a victim. Constant, nagging insults to good sense even-tually wear on the steel of the soul. Logic that flies in the face of logic can madden one. In the years I've spent with Adam, I have learned more about my limits than I ever wanted to know. And yet, in spite of the ridiculous arguments, the life-and-death battles over medication and the puny and wearying orders one must give every day, in spite of pulling gloves onto the chapped, frost-bitten hands of a nearly grown man and knowing he will shed them, once out of sight, in the minus thirty windchill of January, something mysterious has flourished between us, a bond of absolute simplicity, love. That is, unquestionably, the alpha and omega of our relationship, even now that Adam has graduated to a somewhat more independent life.

But as I said, that love is inextricable from anger, and in loving Adam, the anger is mostly directed elsewhere, for it is impossible to love the sweetness, the inner light, the qualities that I trust in Adam, without hating the fact that he will always be kept from fully expressing those aspects of himself because of his biological mother's drinking.

He'll always, all his life, be a lonely person.

I drank hard in my twenties, and eventually got hepatitis. I was lucky. Beyond an occasional glass of wine, I can't tolerate liquor anymore. But from those early days, I understand the urge for alcohol, its physical pull. I had formed an emotional bond with a special configuration of chemicals, and I realize to this day the attraction of the relationship and the immense difficulty in abandoning it.

Adam's mother never let it go. She died of alcohol poisoning, and I'd feel sorrier for her, if we didn't have Adam. As it is, I only hope that she died before she had a chance to produce another child with his problems. I can't help but wish, too, that during her pregnancy, if she couldn't be counseled or helped, she had been forced to abstain for those crucial nine months. On some reservations, the situation has grown so desperate that a jail sentence during pregnancy has been the only answer possible in some cases. Some people have taken more drastic stands and even called for the forced sterilization of women who, after having previously blunted the lives of several children like Adam, refuse to stop drinking while they're pregnant. This will outrage some women, and men, good people who believe that it is the right of the individual to put themselves in harm's way, that drinking is a choice we make, that the individual's liberty to court either happiness or despair is sacrosanct. I believed this, too, and yet the poignancy and frustration of Adam's life has fed my doubts, has convinced me that some of my principles were smug, untested. After all, where is the measure of responsibility here? Where, exactly, is the demarcation between self-harm and child abuse? Gross negligence is nearly equal to intentional wrong, goes a legal maxim. Where do we draw the line?

The people who advocate forcing pregnant women to abstain from drinking come from within the communities dealing with a problem of nightmarish proportions. Still, this is very shaky ground. Once a woman decides to carry a child to term, to produce another human being, has she also the right to inflict on that person Adam's life? Because his mother drank, Adam is one of the earth's damaged. Did she have the right to take away Adam's curiosity, the right to take away the joy he could have felt at receiving a high math score, in reading a book, in wondering at the complexity and quirks of nature? Did she have the right to make him an outcast among children, to make him friendless, to make of his sexuality a problem more than a pleasure, to slit his brain, to give him violent seizures?

It seems to me, in the end, that she had no right to inflict such harm, even from the depth of her own ignorance. Roman Catholicism defines two kinds of ignorance, vincible and invincible. Invincible ignorance is that state in which a person is unexposed to certain forms of knowledge. The other type of ignorance, vincible, is willed. It is a conscious turning away from truth. In either case, I don't think Adam's mother had the right to harm her, and our, son.

Knowing what I know now, I am sure that even when I drank hard I would rather have been incarcerated for nine months and produce a normal child, than bear a human being who would, for the rest of his or her life, be imprisoned by what I did.

And for those still outraged at this position, those so sure, so secure, I say the same thing I say to those who would not allow a poor woman a safe abortion and yet have not themselves gone to adoption agencies and taken in the unplaceable children, the troubled, the unwanted.

If you don't agree with me, then please, go and sit beside the alcohol-affected while they try to learn how to add. My mother, Rita Gourneau Erdrich, who works with disabled children at the Wahpeton Indian School, does this every day. Dry their frustrated tears. Fight for them in the society they don't understand. Tell them every simple thing they must know for survival, one million, two million, three million times. Hold their heads when they have unnecessary seizures and wipe the blood from their bitten lips. Force them to take medicine. Keep the damaged of the earth safe. Love them. Watch them grow up to sink into the easy mud of alcohol. Suffer a crime they commit without remorse or pity. Try and understand lack of conscience. For some, that is the part of the brain and personality affected. And it is horrifying, inexcusable, and most shameful of all, preventable. As taxpayers, you are already paying for their jail terms, and footing the bills for expensive treatment and education. Be a victim yourself, beat your head against a world of brick, fail constantly. Then go back to the mother and father, face to face, and say again: "It was your right."

When I am angriest, I mentally tear into Adam's parents. When I am saddest, I wish them, exhaustedly . . . but there is nowhere to wish them worse than the probable hell of their life and death. And yet, if I ever met Adam's mother, I don't know what I'd do. Perhaps the two of us women would be resigned before this enormous lesson. It is almost impossible to hold another person responsible for so much hurt, even though I know our son was half-starved, tied to the bars of his crib, removed by a welfare agency. In public, when asked to comment on Native American issues, I am defensive. Yes, I say, there are terrible problems. It takes a long, long time to heal communities beaten by waves of conquest and disease. It takes a long time for people to heal themselves. Sometimes, it seems hopeless. Yet in places, it is happening. Tribal communities, most notably the Alkali Lake Band in Canada, are coming together, rejecting alcohol, re-embracing their own humanity, their own culture. These are tough people and they teach a valuable lesson: to whatever extent we can, we must take charge of our lives.

Yet, in loving Adam, we bow to fate. Few of his problems can be solved or ultimately changed. So instead, Michael and I concentrate on only what we can control—our own reactions. If we can muster grace, joy, happiness in helping him confront and conquer the difficulties life presents . . . then we have received gifts. Adam has been deprived of giving so much else.

What I know my husband hopes for, in offering *The Broken Cord*, is a future in which this particular and preventable tragedy will not exist. I feel the same way. Michael and I have a picture of our son. For some reason, in this photograph, taken on my grandfather's land in the Turtle Mountains of North Dakota, no defect is evident in Adam's stance or face. Although perhaps a knowing doctor could make the FAS diagnosis from his features, Adam's expression is intelligent and serene. He is smiling. His eyes are brilliant and his brows are dark, sleek. There is no sign in this portrait that anything is lacking.

I look at this picture and think, "Here is the other Adam. The one our son would be if not for alcohol." Sometimes Michael and I imagine that we greet him, that we look into his eyes, and he into ours, for a long time and in that gaze we not only understand our son, but he also understands us. He has grown up to be a colleague, an equal, not a person who needs pity, protection, or special breaks. By the old reservation cabin where my mother was born, in front of the swirled wheat fields and woods of ancestral land, Adam stands expectantly, the full-hearted man he was meant to be. The world opens before him—so many doors, so much light. In this picture, he is ready to go forward with his life.

CAROL AUSTIN

Latent Tendencies and Covert Acts

We have a little girl available for adoption in Peru. She's four days old. Are you interested?"

Were we interested? "Yes! Yes! Yes!" we screamed with delight, hugging each other and crying tears of joy and disbelief as we turned circles in our kitchen. But suddenly I felt a shadow creeping over me, a warning to hold my joy in check.

You see, the phone call we'd been daring to hope would come, wasn't a call to Jane *and* me. It was a call to my partner, Jane. The adoption agency didn't know I existed.

It was July of 1986 when we decided to pursue a South American adoption. We knew from the beginning that wanting to parent far outweighed our need to test the North Carolina legal system. We didn't think we would get very far if we both tried to adopt the same child. Even now, almost ten years later, as proven parents of very typical seven- and eight-year-olds, we might *still* be denied joint parenting status or even the right to be a lesbian single parent by this not-so-blind judicial system if we decided to go public.

Making the decision to temporarily move our relationship into the closet in order to legally adopt our first daughter was not easy. Both in our forties, each of us had been politically active lesbians since the 1970s. Going back in the closet was a ludicrous notion neither of us thought we would ever again contemplate. However, it was clear, from all we had read and from informal conversations with adoption workers, that to adopt through state or private agencies in 1986, one of us would have to deny her lesbian identity and our relationship in front of the network of agencies, social workers, lawyers, courts and other government officials. The other would have to "disappear." This would be the *real* price of our adoption.

Once we had agreed to take the chance to adopt, determining which one of us would become invisible was an easier decision. Jane was, and still is, a well-established, respected professional, and at the time, I had lived in town for only eighteen months and was still searching for work that I liked and would pay me a decent salary. It made sense for me to become the legally unseen. I assured Jane and convinced myself that my temporary status as the nonexistent mom would be no problem. What a joke.

Five years earlier, Jane had registered with the state to adopt an infant. But as a single person, she had never been offered a child. Then we heard that a single woman friend of Jane's had just adopted an infant from Chile after only a five-month wait.

Jane began making the contact calls and gathering information about various agencies and countries that would allow a single forty-year-old woman to adopt an infant. A few Latin American countries, it turned out, would actually consider her application.

Before moving ahead, Jane and I had endless discussions about the consequences of taking a child out of her birth-culture. For hours we raked the same piece of our souls as we talked about the pain a child might feel not growing up in her birth-culture and perhaps never feeling a part of our Euro-American culture either. We also despised and rejected the view that we might appear to be benevolent white rescuers to a certain segment of the population; a view I'm sure we must present to some people when parts or all of our family wander through a supermarket or other public place.

Soon Jane was traipsing the countryside, attending endless agency adoptive-parent meetings. It was she who could talk animatedly to curious friends and family about our paperwork progress or share the agency anecdotes. My lack of firsthand information made me feel inadequate even when I tried talking about the process to my own friends. Desperately wanting to immerse myself in at least these secondhand details, I listened eagerly and created faces to match the names of people I would never meet. But when the social workers came to interview Jane and look through our home, any obvious signs of me had disappeared. Any messages on our answering machine from the adoption agency were, left, of course, solely for Jane.

I soon found myself emotionally stranded between anger and guilt. I felt angry and totally left out by my externally forced, yet self-imposed, invisibility. And right on the heels of my anger came my guilt! It was, after all, Jane who was putting in all of the hours of meeting time, and it was her financial and personal history that was being dissected. I didn't envy her, yet I began to have an all-or-nothing reaction. I stopped even trying to help Jane deal with all the endless facts and figures the agency needed. Making copies of documents became my only level of involvement. Finally, immersion at *any* level, without any recognition of my existence, became impossible. How naive I had been to assume, only a few months before, that my invisibility would be no problem. The entire adoption situation had forced open some of my raw childhood wounds.

It was 1945. Separating from my father while she was still pregnant with me, my mother soon became a single parent of three in war-ravaged England. Reeling with this predicament, she placed me, an eighteen-month-old baby, in a foster home, sent my eight-year-old brother back to Scotland to live with our birth father and kept my four-year-old sister with her. I didn't live with or even see my mother again until I was almost five. From then on I lived in absolute poverty, in an environment filled with physical and sexual abuse and neglect.

My birth father never saw me after I was born, nor has he laid eyes on me to this day. I met my brother again when I was eleven and have seen him only twice since then. I assume he's still in England, though I have no idea where.

When I was thirteen my mother married an American serviceman. The year before this second marriage, she made an unusual trip to Edinburgh. "Do you know where your mother is now?" my grandmother asked me in her deep Scottish accent. "Getting a divorce from your father, John."

I stood paralyzed by shock, but not about the divorce. My sister had always told me my father was dead, and my mother had never even uttered his name. So, at the age of thirteen, I learned that my father was alive and that his name was John.

A year later, my stepfather legally adopted my sister and me, and we all moved to the United States. My mother, glad to turn her back on years of struggle and suffering, was only too glad to leave England. Although I never spoke about my sadness, my heart ached as I wiped my silent good-bye tears on the fur of my beloved tabby cat, Twinkle. Now—forty years later—the invisible child was volunteering to become an invisible mom. No problem?

After the call from the agency and once Jane and I came back down to earth, we updated our shots, found a housesitter, made plane reservations to Lima, bought a crib and a changing table and interviewed pediatricians to find one who could handle *two* completely involved moms. Our preoccupation with our tasks gave me a three-week reprieve from my fears about becoming the parent-anonymous once we arrived in Peru. I was entirely caught up in the excitement of our imaginings!

Our adoption agency estimated a four-week stay in Lima while the official adoption process took place. Julie, our Peruvian contact, called to tell us the courts and health workers were out on strike. An odd phenomenon to us at the time, but one which became all too familiar during our stay in Peru.

Jane and Julie spoke several times before we left, and I, listening in on each call, began to feel a deepening excitement and amazement at what was happening. Over a crackling phone line, Julie said the baby girl had not yet been officially named, and asked what name to put on the birth certificate. Jane told her, "Catherine," the name we had chosen for our daughter.

We packed a minimal amount of clothing for ourselves, many more clothes for Catherine, and two suitcases plus an army-green duffle bag of diapers and formula, having been told supplies of formula and disposable diapers were either nonexistent or, at the very least, unpredictable. Somehow, and seemingly suddenly, everything fell into place at home and in Peru, and to our utter amazement, we climbed aboard a plane heading for Lima.

During the flight, Jane and I wondered silently and out loud what in the world we were doing flying off to a South American country neither one of us had even thought much about before the phone call. Since that call, we had bought every book on Peru we could find, including a backpacker's guide to the Andes!

Once through Peruvian customs and out of the airport, we stuffed our luggage into the standard Peruvian Volkswagen taxi and headed for Julie's home address where we would live for the coming weeks. Julie, hearing our taxi, was waiting for us at her front door inside a wrought iron and brick fence on the quiet, geranium-lined street. As I stood in the road by our bags, watching the taxi drive off, I silently became invisible once more.

Julie, a forty-year-old American missionary, hugged us hello and, in an emotionally numbing moment for us both, Jane introduced me as her good friend. Immediately Julie asked if Jane wanted to meet her daughter. Of course we did! We quickly threw our baggage into our apartment attached to the side of Julie's house and piled into her beat-up green Jeep.

Dodging cars and pedestrians, we raced through the city's back streets on our way to the family who had been caring for four-week-old Catherine. With my not knowing Spanish, all of the excited conversation between Julie and the foster mother, Anna, sounded rapid and frantic. But Anna was beaming as she disappeared into the back of the house and reappeared carrying an incredibly beautiful, brown-skinned baby wrapped in a crocheted pink blanket. On top of her enormous mop of shiny black hair perched a matching pink hat. Jane and I were dumbfounded. She was more than either of us could absorb in the moment.

Anna carefully handed Catherine to Jane. I took pictures of my speechless, amazed partner while she held her new baby. Jane then handed Catherine to me, and I gently cradled my gorgeous daughter. I was acutely aware that I shouldn't hold her forever, because, after all, as far as all these strangers were concerned, this was the daughter for whom *only* Jane had been waiting a very long time. Julie glowed, and Anna smiled happily and nodded.

Our four-week stay in Peru extended to seven weeks as striking workers kept closing and opening government offices. We traveled to Machu Picchu, the lost city of the Incas, and to Lake Titicaca, the highest navigable lake in the world, where people live on floating reed islands they weave and repair themselves, but most of our time was spent in Lima. Roaming the noisy city with our new month-old daughter tucked down in her baby pack against one of our chests, we would head downtown about ten-thirty each morning, eat lunch in the same little restaurant and walk through the streets and shops until almost dark. We ate some meals with Julie, her jovial husband Will, an engineer, and their three teenage sons. But days away from Julie's house were our time, time when we didn't have to pretend we were anything other than a brand new family.

A real joy for us was being able to spend a lot of time with Catherine's birth mother, Violetta, a twenty-two-year-old Quechua Indian who was also Julie's maid. When Violetta had become pregnant out of wedlock, she had been taken in by some distant family members who struggled to care for their own five children. Living in a crowded, dirt-floored home in a poverty-ridden neighborhood in Lima, the family was not willing to care for another child. And if Violetta decided to keep her child, she could not work. Violetta's and her child's survival depended upon her giving up this first-born baby to adoption.

Because of my own spotty family history, using one of Julie's sons as our interpreter, I gathered as much information about Catherine's heritage as I could. We took many pictures of Violetta, including profiles, so Catherine could later see where she got her nose and her gorgeous smile. With charade-like gestures and Jane's college Spanish, we soon found ourselves laughing a great deal, the three of us openly sharing our deep love, amazement and laughter as we hovered over little Catherine. We were three women with whom this child, for better or worse, was forever connected.

As lawyers, courts, Julie, Catherine's foster family and the American consulate staff concentrated their energy on Jane, Catherine's new mother, I instinctively put my energy into connecting with my new daughter. It was a good way to survive these official and painful times.

When we went to court, Jane would have to take Catherine down rabbit-warren hallways to listen to lawyers and judges and I would wait for hours in cream-colored rooms with exposed pipes, peeling paint and disinterested military-attired clerks, who talked and laughed endlessly on their black dial telephones.

Outside of court, however, I took over the bulk of the holding and carrying time with our new daughter, while Jane struggled between meeting her own need to connect with Catherine and trying to assuage my feelings of invisibility. It was a difficult daily balance for her, and I didn't make it any easier, because I couldn't seem to raise myself out of the mire of feeling overlooked, unimportant and invisible at every turn.

I soon became Catherine's main mom, and by the time we returned to the States, Jane had begun to feel the pain of being invisible to our daughter. Intellectually I knew that I had to begin sharing this mother-role with Jane, but it was a real emotional adjustment on my part.

Family and friends welcomed us home, but again, because I was a relative newcomer to Jane's environment, I still felt twinges of being the invisible mom or being second-best when people would make an enormous fuss over Jane. They certainly included me in their joy, but these were, after all, mostly Jane's friends, who had known her for ten-plus years. Jane's large family also poured excitement on us from all directions.

Years earlier, my mother had stopped talking to me when I told her I was a lesbian. She knew, through my sister, that Jane and I had gone to Peru and she told my sister that I would make a good parent, but I never heard from her or my stepfather. (My mother died in 1991, and although I sent pictures, she never set eyes on her Peruvian-born grandchildren or her incredible daughter-in-law.) Thankfully, my sister, her husband and their three children came and stayed for a week to welcome Catherine home.

Our second call came directly from a woman lawyer in Lima in early autumn 1988. "I am holding a gorgeous eight-month-old little girl. She's available for adoption. Are you interested?" Were we interested? "Yes! Yes! Yes!" we screamed, once again hugging each other, shedding tears of joy and delight as we turned circles in our kitchen. Catherine was fifteen-months-old, and we had decided to pursue another Peruvian adoption. This time there was no shadow of fear clouding my celebration. I already had the security of Catherine's love to lessen the dread of my impending invisibility once we reached Peru again.

For this second adoption, Jane's background checks simply needed updating since our shots and passports were all in order. Jane flew to Lima the first week in October and met our second daughter, whom we named Victoria. Because of my work schedule, I brought Catherine a week later. After a cancelled flight in Miami and losing our luggage because of it, our family of four finally met in the back of a taxi at midnight. A tired but totally captivating eight-month-old girl squinted at me and her new big sister through the hazy blue glow of the streetlights.

Then she snuggled her head back into Jane's neck and fell asleep.

This time we were prepared for a seven-week stay in Lima and rented our own apartment. But Peru was a scarier place now, with the Shining Path guerrillas blowing up hydroelectric plants, leaving the capital city with sporadic water and electricity, and closing shops. During one courthouse visit, Jane and Victoria ended up under a desk in a clerk's office as they listened to people running, yelling and shooting in the hallway.

With two active toddlers and concerned about safety, we decided not to travel outside of Lima and again spent an enormous amount of time walking the bustling streets. Within the security of our apartment, we celebrated our joy of being a family.

After having spent a full week alone with Jane in Lima, little Victoria was completely attached to her new mother and not at all interested in having a *second* devoted mom. She tolerated me when Jane was around, but if Jane left, Victoria would scream bloody murder. Victoria, it seemed, could take only one person at a time into her heart, and Jane was that person for a very long time.

Today Victoria and I have a wonderful relationship; her personality, in fact, is enough like mine to make Jane and me laugh. Nevertheless, from the very beginning, up to the present day, if either of the girls becomes scared or sick, each seems to reach for the mom with whom she first bonded.

After our family returned home with baby Victoria, my invisibility issue again began to raise its ugly head. We had always agreed that Jane should re-adopt both Catherine and Victoria through the U.S. courts. And although I didn't have to physically disappear during this paper-pushing transaction, the existence of yet more legal documents that ignored my presence as the girls' mother made me feel awful. Any feelings of inferiority or inadequacy tucked away inside me again appeared. I felt as if I were being scolded by a critical parent who kept reminding me of my rightful place!

Even now, after eight years of being a mom, I find myself incredibly sensitive to the slightest inference that I may not be the girls' "real" mother. For example, if people talk more to Jane than to me about our kids, I can still begin to emotionally drop out of the conversation. It doesn't matter that some of these people don't even know our legal adoptive circumstance, my paranoia still kicks in, and I feel myself begin to evaporate right under my own nose. In an instant, I find myself believing our girls *really* are Jane's because the law says so! For example, if Jane and I fight, and I decide she would rather I leave—not that she has *ever* indicated that—I envision myself moving out and become heartsick imagining how I would live without my children.

The four of us also deal with another kind of invisibility . . . being a two-parent lesbian family in an ever-so-heterosexual world. Whether it's accurate or not, this majority culture seems to slot the mother as the primary parent. Given that our daughters have *two* primary parents, Jane and I have put a lot of effort into helping our daughters take their atypical family in stride.

For example, we never let our daughters hear either of us deny she is our child. This means that in grocery stores, on playgrounds and at camp-grounds, we often startle people by both answering yes when one of us is asked, "And is this beautiful little girl your daughter?"

Only too well do I remember my own maternal confusion when I was four years old: I had climbed onto a double-decker bus ahead of my foster mother, Aunt Kit, but the bus started to pull away before she was safely on. She fell and was dragged several feet before the frantic conductor got the driver to stop. Not immediately aware of what was going on, I found myself being hurriedly ushered by adult hands down the aisle away from the scene. At some point I realized that all of the commotion and chaos meant some-thing was very wrong with Aunt Kit. I began trying to scramble back. Adults stopped me and told me everything was all right. One woman, firmly block-ing my way, asked, "Is that your mummy, dear?" In my heart I paused, momentarily confused, because I knew she wasn't, but I didn't know who was. However, I obviously knew the power of the "mummy" connection, so through my scared four-year-old tears, I blubbered a yes.

Jane and I have individual wills that we hope will protect our family. They are written in a way that completely ignores the fact that I have no legal standing as my daughters' mother. If either of us dies, both of our wills name the other person as the sole parent to our daughters. If both of us die, we have appointed legal guardians. We do not have any agreement about what we would do if we were to separate.

Very few family members or friends know whether one of us adopted both children or if each of us adopted a child. We firmly believe that this information colors the filter through which people view our family. Shortly after we returned home, we were at a lesbian-parent gathering when an adoptive parent, obviously struggling with the invisibility issue herself, asked us, "But who's their *real* mother?" We never told her what she really wanted to know.

Both daughters have our last names joined with a hyphen. That is the way their family name is written on their birth certificates and how we've always used it. Our children call Jane "Mother" and me "Mamma." They have never had any trouble remembering what to call us, and in restaurants they can make heads turn, when in their loud voices they proclaim, "Mother, Mamma, guess what?"

Jane and I fully realize that we can no longer choose when to be out. As lesbian parents, in a biracial family, we are visible wherever we go, whether it's simply in our neighborhood or searching out day care, schools, religious communities, doctors, dentists, music teachers and so on. We present ourselves as out, same-gender parents trying to pave the way ahead of our daughters. At school, Jane is active on several committees and has given several diversity workshops for the teachers and staff. I write a monthly column for the girls' school newspaper with an author's blurb saying that Jane and I parent Catherine and Victoria.

Jane and I are ever-present moms. Our daughters do not experience one laid-back, less-than-hands-on parent. A friend told us we reminded her of a comment Woody Allen made in one of his movies after he had apparently lost his wife to a female partner and she had taken their child. He told his friend that he had barely survived one mother, how was his child to survive *two?*

Recently, we have been dealing with our eight-year-old's feelings of pain around being adopted. Both of us sit and talk to her about the "Why didn't she want me?" question. Her school friends really complicate the issue when they ask her who her *real* mother is!

Jane and I often chuckle, saying that we have given our brown-skinned daughters built-in therapy issues: adoption, a biracial family in a predominantly white North Carolina culture and lesbian parents! But we also see these realities as real family strengths. Together we are learning how to "world-travel"—to comfortably move in and out of other people's worlds— to value different family structures and to celebrate the joy of diversity.

SUSAN WADIA-ELLS

The Anil Journals

I am one-eighth Asian Indian and proud of this heritage—my curly Parsi hair and intense eyes—and of my mother's family, the Wadias, still one of the most respected Parsi families in India As a child growing up in Vineland, New Jersey, I had tried to impress my third grade classmates by speaking "Indian" which I convinced them I was fluent in because my grandmother was half Asian Indian I also visited India a number of times as a young adult where I often felt as if I had finally come home. Sometimes I could see my grandmother's generous nose, her olive skin and dark penetrating eyes, or the color and texture of my mother's thick hair in the people around me.

In 1985 I was thirty nine years old, just married, and unwilling to take any surgical steps to deal with my apparent infertility. I wanted to be a mother, not a medical case. So my life-partner, Larry, and I agreed that we would adopt a child. Larry had never thought about adoption before, let alone the question of where to adopt from. I had always wanted to adopt a child someday. Now that my "someday" had arrived, I wanted to adopt a child from India.

Larry and I applied to the Vermont Children's Aid Society, an adoption agency with an ongoing relationship with the large Calcutta-based International Mission of Hope. The agency said we would most likely receive an infant boy because we were a married couple and most of the many single-women applying to adopt children from IMH were requesting girls. Soon Larry and I were happily arguing about a name for our forthcoming baby boy.

"He'll need an Indian name," I insisted. "He's Indian, damn it!"

"He's already Indian. He'll need an American name. He's going to live in

America," was my partner's retort.

For some reason Larry thought that "Alysandyr" sounded American. "We can call him Alex for short," he said.

"Never," I vowed silently to myself. "This child's name is Anil."

Anil, a popular Indian name that means "fresh air" or "wind" in the Hindi language of northern Indian and "blue sky" in the Bengali language of eastern India, sounded just right to my heart. So in the end, months before any baby was born, we sent off his stack of immigration and adoption papers with a name that was surely longer than the baby himself. "Alysandyr Anil Wadia-Nevin."

A year later when the baby was two months old and legally could be "assigned" to a non-Indian family, we received a note written in English, that was included in the envelope with our baby's first picture.

"Alysandyr Anil is a handsome little boy as you can see in the photo taken a while back. His nursery name is Anil. It was strange to see that you have also named him Anil."

Who are we to think that we can decide such things as a child's name? I suppose his Bengali nurse and I each chose the name "Anil," not because we liked it better than any other Indian name, but because this was the child's name. Born into a world where his birth mother had to leave him behind, this child, with those eyes that look and smile and miss nothing, knows himself very well. Possibly he is here to teach, more than to learn.

October 28, 1986, India's largest festival, Diwali, the festival of lights, was just a few days away. Diwali is the happiest holy day of the Hindu calendar and the beginning of India's spiritual year, surely auspicious signs for me as I moved closer and closer toward motherhood.

As the train's ancient coal engine barreled through the northeastern state of Bihar, all I could think of, looking out at the red tile roofs and glistening black water buffalo wandering near the rice paddies, was that by the end of the day I would have my baby in my arms. I would be a mom.

When the Rajvani Express finally pulled into Calcutta's Howrah Station at 9 A.M., the ragged, cavernous building was teeming with coolies, *sadhus*, mangy dogs, encamped families, fellow travelers, holy cows and soda sellers. At that moment, Calcutta seemed the most beautiful city in the world to me. Larry was not so sure.

A taxi driver saw us—two pink-faced Americans with backpacks—emerge from the station entrance and quickly herded us, along with a tall, middle-aged Indian man with a protruding nose and a faded brown briefcase, into his small, battered Ambassador taxi cab. Packed into the sedan, we lurched forward toward the chaotic mass of traffic slowly moving onto the bridge to downtown Calcutta. It wasn't long before we came to a full stop.

The beak-nosed "professor" lectured us as we sat knee-to-knee waiting for traffic around us to move: "Here in Calcutta, people are all right until they're asked to work. Democracy without education. In America, time is costly. Here people can wait two hours on a trolley, no problem. In Calcutta, time is the cheapest thing."

Finally, the mass of traffic trembled and our cab began to inch onto India's Golden Gate, the infamous Howrah Bridge, spanning the Hooghly River and carrying passengers between the immense Howrah train station and India's largest city.

"Keep your arm inside. The car can get bumped," the professor barked at me. "This you can see nowhere in the world. Not Bombay, not Delhi, only Calcutta," he continued.

Lines of trolley cars, circa 1940, ran down the middle of the bridge, right alongside our car. People perched on the trolleys' glassless window ledges, dangling their legs in the traffic, while other brave—or foolish—souls squatted on the trolleys' roofs. A few rickshaws, along with bicycles, motor scooters and three-wheeled diesel "phut-phuts," kept trying to squeeze between us and the trolleys. Ahead I could see more black and yellow Ambassador taxis scattered among huge dump trucks adorned with colorful murals of Hindu gods, landscapes and decorative Bengali script. As we sat in the middle of this Calcutta beehive, the "professor" still venting his frustration with his culture and his fellow countrymen, I smiled, dreaming about my sleeping baby on the other side of town.

When the cab finally inched off the bridge an hour later, we started down a road lined with tall office buildings. Large sections of the pavement were buckled and a broken fire hydrant sprayed gallons of water into the street while skinny children and sharp-boned silver-grey cows waded back and forth in the mud enjoying the festivities. "That's a Calcutta monsoon flood," the professor said, finally drawing some humor from the swirling city scene.

At the hotel, an old British woman behind the reception desk gave me a good map. Tollygunge Circular Road, a short semicircle of a street, would be a cinch to find. But finding the International Mission of Hope, at 35/6 Tollygunge Circular Road, turned out to be another story. Back and forth we went. The street numbers jumping from 77/8 to 25/6 to 124/5 without notice, around and around, up and down. The driver finally forgot about numbers and started asking for the place for the babies, for IMH, or for what he thought might be the Bengali translation of IMH. On our fourth try down the quiet narrow residential street scattered with stalls selling juice or the spicy betel-nut pan, sandal fixers, spice merchants and a few small temples, my searching eyes caught a white flash in the sun—a tall, enclosed Jeep, enamel white, with clear black English letters along its side: *International Mission of Hope.*

"It's IMH!!" I screamed as I scrambled out of the taxi and hurried toward a beautiful woman in a blue-and-white-striped cotton sari standing by a door in the heavy sunlight. Larry paid the driver and caught up with me and to-gether we followed the smiling woman into the cool cement building.

No introductions were needed. The nursery staff was waiting for us. We had been sending four-month-old Anil postcards every day telling him we had arrived in India.

Another woman wearing the same IMH cotton sari pointed to a chubby figure sitting on the lap of a woman on the opposite side of the clean, cool room. The nursery was lined wall to wall with sleeping babies in bassinets or held by nurses, while a few larger babies slept peacefully on mats laid in the middle of the floor.

As I began to walk across the still room toward Anil, careful not to trample the sleeping infants, the women holding other babies along the sides of the room began to quietly chant "mother, mother, mother."

Anil knew me immediately as I knelt on the floor and clucked to him. He opened up his big eyes even wider, and a grin broke out on his face.

"That's my Anil," I murmured, as I took him gently and held him close. The tears I had been holding back as I traveled across half of the world's oceans, rivers and roads to reach my son now bathed my face and dripped on his little nose, dissolving us into one big hug.

"That's not our baby," Larry blurted out. "Our baby is not this fat."

The round-faced cherub who now filled my arms stopped smiling and glared at his new father.

"Larry, don't be silly, look at his eyes! He's gained a lot of weight since his picture was taken a few months ago," I whispered as I too glared at this new father who stood beside me. For many weeks, while Anil was busy doubling his birthweight, Larry and I had carried around copies of our one and only photo of Anil, a skinny two-week-old, six- or seven-pound infant. As new parents, we would constantly stare adoringly at this picture of our thin-cheeked baby's face, a face now imprinted in Larry's brain.

During that eventful October day in Calcutta, while my passion remained focused on Anil, my child, I also felt a nagging curiosity about the woman who had given birth to him a few months earlier. Who was she? How had she become pregnant? Why had she decided to give up Anil at his birth? What was she feeling right now about her decision? Would I ever be able to find her, to thank her for this incredible gift? Intellectually I knew that these questions were probably unanswerable, but without the ability to thank her, the whole adoption felt somewhat surreal. How can you have a birth without a birth mother?

Before even applying for the adoption, I had been told that the International Mission of Hope orphanage received babies who had been abandoned by their birth mothers. These women were unwed mothers, or widows we were told. It was socially unacceptable for them to even become pregnant. As our adoption papers were processed, IMH had continued to make it stridently clear that no records of the birth parents would be available for these children or even existed.

When I asked the IMH director if we might meet the doctor who had delivered Anil, she suggested that Larry and I accompany their staff member, Besanti, the next morning as she made her daily rounds of the "nursing homes." These nursing homes—doctors' offices containing a few hospital beds—are found throughout India.

So the next day, while Anil took his long morning nap at IMH with his beloved nurse, Koshal-lal, nearby, Larry and I followed Besanti into a waiting vehicle. On the way, the driver jumped out at his favorite pan stall, hopping back into the black IMH Ambassador sedan a minute later with two packed banana leaves in hand. He passed one spicy pan to Besanti and offered the other to Larry, who politely declined. The driver popped the second pan in his mouth and, slowly chewing the concoction of red-staining betel nut and spices, moved on into the swirl of downtown Calcutta traffic.

When we stopped by Sri Krishna Nursing Home, where Anil had been born, Besanti and I found Dr. Chakraborty sitting at his desk in the second-floor suite of rooms. First I humbly thanked the tall, grey-haired doctor for delivering my child. Then I asked, "Can you tell me about the mothers who give birth to their babies and then leave them?"

"All of the women who come here are very, very poor," Dr. Chakraborty said in his clipped Indian English. "Some of them have four, five, six children already; they may not even have a home. They cannot keep more children. I am happy though to give the children to IMH. I have been to your country three times escorting babies. I see how very well cared for these children are. They are quite strong."

Back in the IMH sedan, now stuck in a mid-morning Calcutta traffic jam, Besanti held our first baby of the morning up into the warm sunlight streaming through the car's side window.

"Who are these mothers?" I asked Besanti, as we drove toward yet another nursing home to pick up one or two more waiting newborn babies. Besanti heard my question and gave me a startled look.

"They are not mothers," Besanti said quickly, then lowered her dark eyes and the tiny baby as we moved slowly forward in the line of traffic.

"We rarely see babies who are over three pounds," Cheri Clark, an American nurse and founder of the IMH orphanage, told us later that day. "The doctors who run these little nursing homes used to leave the newborns on the floor until they died. But we have gone round to each of their offices and given them 'space blankets' to cover the children. They know we will come to their offices each day to pick up any babies who have been abandoned. Most of the doctors are using these feather-weight insulated blankets now. It's good. Now the babies are alive when we arrive to pick them up."

I nodded mutely, barely hearing her words. There was so much about India I didn't understand.

Tomorrow Larry and I would bundle up Anil, pick up his white canvas IMH bag filled with tiny shirts, sleepers, diapers, wipes and formula and fly west out of Calcutta to Bombay and Vermont beyond. But first Koshal-lal and the other women who had nurtured Anil for the past four months needed to say their good-byes.

"Tell them they are one with the angels," Larry said to Cheri Clark the next day, as Koshal-lal and many of the other *masseys* (Bengali for "mother's elder sister"), stood at the gate waving and wiping tears from their eyes. Larry, his face wet from his own tears, gently carried his son, now sleeping peacefully in his wicker travel basket, into the waiting Ambassador cab. Our grey-bearded Sikh driver, tall in his red turban, stood holding the door while I snapped pictures of everyone in sight. We were all part of Anil's ongoing birth story, his second or third delivery of sorts, I figured. Looking at my calm, sleeping baby, I suddenly wondered how many lives this child had already had.

A few years later, on Anil's fourth birthday, he and I made his birthday cake: angel food cake, stuffed with chocolate pudding and whipped cream and frosted with more whipped cream and topped with chocolate shavings.

Later we talked about how four years earlier, when it had been time for Anil to be born, he had slid right out of his birth mother's "bagina." I said, "She looked down and saw it was you, and she said, 'Oh, look, it's Anil! It's Anil!' and she quickly called your *massey*, your nurse, Koshal-lal. 'Koshal-lal, please—Anil is here! Please call Larry and Susie to come to Calcutta now!

Anil is born!'" I retold Anil's birth fable to him for the seventy-fifth time.

"So Koshal-lal called us, and we were so excited. We screamed. We cried. I shouted at Larry, 'Don't be your usual slow-poke self. Get packed up, come on, we have to go to India now!' We got on a huge airplane, and we flew and we flew and we flew across the Atlantic Ocean and the Indian Ocean until we got to Bombay, and then we went by train to Calcutta and you.

"Meanwhile Koshal-lal was taking such good, good care of you. She sang to you every day: 'Oh-nil; Oh-nil.' She would even hold you while you were taking your afternoon nap. And if she dared to put you down—boy would you scream. 'Please carry me for my *whole* afternoon nap!' you would say. But when your dad and I arrived, Koshal-lal let Larry carry you outside in the soft Calcutta air for your nap. And then Larry wouldn't put you down either. In fact he carried you across most of the Indian and the Atlantic oceans, because whenever you'd cry, he would gently take you and hold you close, and carry you up and down the aisle of the Air India air bus, and then the aisle of the Pan Am 747, and rock you and sing you back to smiles and sleep."

"What's my birth mom's name?" Anil asked one day, months later.

"I don't know," I told him. "But I really want to know. Anyway we could still give her a name. Your beautiful birth mother needs a name. What name shall we call her?"

"Let's call her Green Popcorn," Anil said with a happy, wide grin.

"Anil! . . . no way," I said. "Your beautiful birth mother needs to have a much nicer name than Green Popcorn."

Anil thought for a moment. "Okay, we can call her Koshal-lal too. Then we'll have two Koshal-lals," he said.

"Oh, good," I said. "Two Koshal-lals."

"And she can come visit us from India and stay for two weeks, and she can sleep on top of the refrigerator," announced Anil with growing gusto.

"Anil!" I said. "She can't sleep on top of the refrigerator. She needs a nice place to sleep."

"Okay, she can sleep in my room while she's here, and I"ll get to 'nuggle' all night with you and Dad," he said.

When it was Anil's fifth birthday we brought in our green and brown relief world globe to Anil's Morningsong Waldorf Preschool. In Morningsong's tradition, the class gathered around the birthday child, as Mrs. Chapman, his teacher, told Anil's birth story. "Five years ago today, Anil sat way high up on a star and looked down. 'Where do I want to be born?' he thought. 'Who do I want my parents to be? I love India . . . look how beautiful the people are. I love the women's saris, the turbans and the *longhi* that the men are wearing. Look at the high Himalaya Mountains, the highest in the whole world. It is gentle down there. I want to go there, where the cows walk slowly through the dusty market streets, where kids eat *japati* and *puri* and lots of rice and *masala dhosa* everyday, where snow sits on the tallest mountain tops all year long. But where are my parents? There they are! But why are Larry and Susie over on the other side of the world in the mountains of Vermont? They need to come to India. I'll go to India. We can all be together soon in India.' "

Then Larry and I showed the class how our plane had flown across the Atlantic and then across the Indian Ocean to Bombay, until we finally reached Anil in Calcutta and flew back together to Vermont. The four- and five-year-old children talked about Anil's intercontinental birth story for days, envious that they had not thought to arrive on the other side of the world, thus making their parents come running to get them at their birth.

Last summer, Josephine, a new friend, chatted with me as we fixed dinner in her rambling old Vermont kitchen. Anil, now eight, played with Josephine's two children, a girl and a boy also adopted from IMH.

"These women, the widows and the unwed teens, deny that they're pregnant," Josephine said. "They can keep their pregnancy hidden under their saris until the seventh or eighth month, but then they begin to show. They have heard about several doctors' offices in certain sections of Calcutta who will induce the birth. So they go."

I sucked in my breath as I heard her words. My mind flew back to 1986 and our baby-gathering trip with Besanti in downtown Calcutta. Suddenly I remembered the second floor of the IMH nursery. Upstairs were the preemie wards—room after room after room filled with "low birth-weight" babies weighing two and three pounds. Mittens covered their hands and their feet and intravenous tubes were taped to their noses so they could receive liquids that their throats could not yet swallow.

"We can't use incubators because the electricity goes off too often. Here if these babies live through the first day, we just hold on to them and don't let them die after that," Cheri Clark had said in her warm but matter-of-fact tone.

Suddenly a space in my mind cleared. Now I understood why many of these babies were not held by a mother's hands immediately after their birth.

Now I understood why some of these infants were held only by space-blankets until Besanti arrived to take them. Was this "saving" an act of human compassion, I wondered, or was this profound cultural arrogance?

From the first photo taken a few weeks after his birth, to our present-day life, Anil has seemed the "old soul" of the three of us. His eyes have always been deep and centered. Never a wild-eyed innocent baby, he has always had a knowing sense about him. Even today at the ripe old age of eight he will sit, looking out at the mountains, stroking his dog, lost in his thoughts for long periods of time.

"How long did it take you to get to India?" he asked me one night recently as we were "nuggling down" to go to sleep.

"You were nineteen weeks old when we arrived in Calcutta."

"What did my birth mom say to Koshal-lal when she gave me to her?"

I realized that it was time to revise Anil's birth fable. "I don't know, but I would love to know," I said. "If I could get to meet your birth mom, I would be so excited and so happy to see her that I would make a mess. I would start to cry and cry and cry and say, 'Thank you. Thank you for giving me Anil to be my baby, because I am lucky to have the bestest baby in the whole world.'"

And Anil said, "No, Mom, you can't say those things. Don't say so: don't brag. How much did I weigh when you got me?" Anil asked, quickly changing the subject.

"Twelve pounds," I said. "You were one of the biggest babies who ever lived at IMH. You were already six pounds when you were born."

"Is my birthday the same day that you and Daddy met me in Calcutta?"

"No," I said. "You were born on June 18 and we got to Calcutta October 28, just before Halloween. Should we celebrate that day?"

"Yes," he said adamantly.

"We'll call it our family birthday, because that's the day we all became a family," I said. "We'll each have two birthdays. That will be nice."

"Yeah," he said, before drifting off to sleep.

WENDY LICHTMAN

Visiting Suzanne

Not long before I took my seven-year-old daughter to Colorado to visit her birth mother, I read one of those studies about twins separated at birth and raised in different homes. How, the researchers wanted to know this time, did environment affect eating patterns? The most problematic eater in the group was a girl whose mother complained that the child wouldn't eat anything that didn't have cinnamon on it—mealtimes were a nightmare. When the researchers interviewed the mother who had raised the other twin, though, they were told that she was a fine eater. "As long as I sprinkle a little cinnamon on her food," the second mother bragged, "she'll eat anything."

There are bonds, I thought, that are beyond our understanding. It's a thought I had often when Bekah and I were in Colorado.

Bekah's birth mother, Suzanne, and I write each other once a year at Bekah's birthday time, sending photos and news, and Suzanne always sends a birthday present. One gift, a handpainted plate with the picture of a young girl that looks a bit like Bekah, became a particular treasure. Bekah kept it in her room, then in the kitchen, then the attic with her baby things, then on the dining room table. She was searching, it seemed, for an area in the house that was special enough, but could never find quite the right place.

Bekah always cried and spoke about missing Suzanne after she got a present, and, on her fifth birthday, when a photo of Suzanne's new baby arrived, she begged to go see them. Someday, I promised her, we would.

When she became literate, Bekah decided that she, too, was going to write Suzanne yearly. In careful printing with purple marker, she wrote her first letter.

Dear Suzanne,

I am 6 now. I can ride a two wheel bike.
This is my first time I lost my tooth.
I want to see my half-sister.

Love Bekah

I had assumed that Bekah would visit her birth mother when she was a teen-ager or a young adult, so I surprised myself when I awoke one summer morning three years ago, turned to my husband and said, "I want to take Bekah to see Suzanne."

The only reason I gave myself then and still give myself now, as to why I made that major decision so easily, was that my close friend was dying of cancer that summer, leaving a four-year-old daughter. That morning my thought process went something like this: Mari is not going to see her daughter grow up and so I must take Bekah to see Suzanne now, before anyone else is dead. It makes sense only in grief, perhaps, and then it makes perfect sense.

I called Suzanne in Colorado Springs that afternoon, and had an awkward conversation with her. She was hesitant to have us visit, concerned especially about two things. One, because Bekah is deaf and primarily uses sign language, Suzanne was worried about how they would communicate. And two, she was scared that Bekah would ask her the hard question: Why did you give me up? I tried to reassure her on both counts. Bekah is used to relating to people who don't sign, and I would be there for interpreting, I explained. If they wanted some private time, I told Suzanne, Bekah was a good reader, so they could write notes. As for the second worry, I really didn't think that question was on Bekah's mind at this time. She tells the birth mother-giving-me-to-my-mom-and-dad story differently each time she tells it, but it always includes the part about Suzanne not being ready to have a family, and us *really* wanting another child, and how brave and generous Suzanne was and how grateful and lucky we were. Trying not to pressure Suzanne, I made up a conference in Denver. If she would like the visit, I told her, I would bring Bekah with me and we could drive to Colorado Springs for a day. Please think about it, I asked.

The next day, she called back and said yes.

Bekah and I spent Friday night in Denver and went to a Mexican restaurant in a pink castle that a friend had told me not to miss. There was a pool of water in the middle of the place that performers dove into during our meal, a dancing gorilla, a magician, a gun fight. Bekah said this was the best vacation of her life.

The ride to Colorado Springs is about an hour, and Bekah, who usually doesn't stop talking and signing, sat silently with a coloring pad and crayons on her lap. We had already talked about the plans; Suzanne was going to meet us at the hotel for the afternoon, then we would have dinner with her husband and Rachelle, Bekah's two-year-old half-sister. We'd spend the night at the hotel, visit with Suzanne's family again the next day, and return to Denver after that. When I asked Bekah how she was doing, she shrugged. When I said the mountains were beautiful, she nodded. For most of the drive Bekah watched her thumbnail scratch a dent into a blue crayon.

And then, finally, after an hour long ride and seven years, Bekah was facing her birth mother. "You are so beautiful," Suzanne whispered. Without sign language interpretation, Bekah understood. She and Suzanne hugged, then Suzanne and I hugged, and then in our nervous excitement, Bekah and I hugged. Suzanne gave Bekah the gift that she said was from her two-year-old; a wonderful stuffed Pooh bear, exactly like the one Rachelle slept with nightly, but one size larger. The day before, Bekah had gone shopping with her father to buy Rachelle a gift and had decided on a soft yellow panda bear exactly like the one she sleeps with, but one size smaller. I tried to contain myself, and to pretend that I believed that a mother and daughter who buy identical presents for their first meeting was only a delightful coincidence. But I believed nothing of the sort. I believed that Suzanne and Bekah were like the twins who ate cinnamon on everything.

Suzanne showed Bekah old photos of herself as a child and of the rest of Bekah's birth family. She knew from our letters that Bekah was studying gymnastics, and she brought along a gymnastics ribbon she had won when she was Bekah's age.

Suzanne had learned the sign language alphabet, and as she shyly tried fingerspelling, Bekah was delighted to correct her and teach her some words. Their private conversation, though, happened on paper. Beneath the flowers and doodles that the two of them had drawn on a piece of our hotel stationery, Suzanne wrote, "Is there anything you want to ask me?"

"One question," Bekah printed. "Okay?"

"Anything is okay," Suzanne answered bravely.

"What," Bekah asked, "is your middle name?"

The next day, I thought about those twins again. I was standing in Suzanne's living room looking at the framed photos of Bekah on the mantel, while Bekah and Rachelle went into the bedroom to change for the pool. When Bekah came out of the room carrying her sister and I saw that Rachelle's bathing suit was the toddler version of the very same wild jungle print material that Bekah had insisted on buying, I gasped. There had been fifty swimsuits on that rack.

"Look at them!" I exclaimed to Suzanne's husband, who thought it merely a cute coincidence, and ran for the camera.

"It's the same material!" I signed hysterically to Bekah, who happily signed back, "Sisters!"

Nobody but me seemed to be flipping out over this thing, so when we got to the pool I found a pay phone and called home, even though I knew nobody would be there at eleven o'clock in the morning. "Now the girls have got matching swim suits on!" I squealed into our answering machine. "Honey, these two kids are *wearing the same bathing suits!!*"

At McDonald's, Suzanne and I talked for an hour while the girls played, and I wondered about our own connection; not quite friends, not quite family. While we spoke intimately about our pasts, our children, our relationships, I tried to figure out what we were to each other.

We all cried when we said good-bye Sunday afternoon, but it wasn't until Bekah got in the car and we pulled away from the apartment that she began to wail—a deep guttural call of pure grief. I pulled over to hold her, but she asked me to please keep driving.

Bekah was ten months old when Suzanne left her at my house, old enough to sob when her mother walked out the door. After a while my son, six at the time, jumped around with a rattle, and Bekah, looking up at her brother for the first time, began to giggle. This time, it was harder. Bekah was still crying miles later when I stopped for gas and cold drinks. When I showed her how to make spit balls from little bits of napkin and shoot them through the straw, she was kind enough to smile at me.

We got to Denver at dinner time and Bekah wanted to go to that goofy restaurant in the pink castle again. It wasn't quite so much fun the second time though, and we were back at the hotel early. Exhausted, Bekah fell asleep next to the Pooh bear and the yellow panda, while I sat with my journal, trying to put my thoughts on paper. Before we came, I hadn't thought that I would feel competitive with Suzanne, in part because of the language barrier between her and Bekah. But I found myself writing about those childhood pictures. When we get home, I decided, I wanted to show Bekah photographs from *my* childhood.

I wrote about the stuffed animals and the bathing suits, of course, but I thought the trip had been so successful not because of the things that seemed extraordinary, but more, in fact, because of the things that seemed ordinary. Suzanne was a person now, not a fairy godmother. Bekah had gone for a swim and had an ice cream cone with her birth mother; she had seen her home, her daughter, her gymnastics ribbon. "I'm so grateful," I wrote, "that I had the courage to come here."

The next morning Bekah and I awoke with energy, took a swim, and then raced to the dining room to get the breakfast that came with the price of our room before it was too late. In the buffet line we noticed a deaf couple sign-ing, and, as the four of us served ourselves, we chatted. Bekah was happy to find other deaf people, and when she finished eating, she went over to their table to visit.

With sign language, it's easy to eavesdrop across tables, and while I fin-ished my coffee I enjoyed watching the conversation. They had just gotten married the day before, the woman told Bekah. Fifty people were at their wedding.

I picked Bekah up from the newlyweds table, wished them well, and we headed out to our car.

"Do you know that at Paul and Sharon's wedding—at their very own wed-ding," Bekah repeated for emphasis, "nobody signed but them?"

"Really?" I asked sadly.

"Yep," Bekah nodded. "Paul said they didn't really understand the service, but he *thinks* they're married." Bekah laughed at Paul's joke and slipped her hand into mine. "They have the honeymoon suite," she explained. "Way up there," she pointed high, in the direction of the outside elevator.

We were at the car already, but Bekah didn't go in the passenger door. Instead, she walked with me to my side. Still holding my hand, she signed with her other one, "Paul and Sharon said I'm lucky you're my mother," she told me.

Bekah liked to wear her hair tied up and over to one side. As I reached down and held her to me, I rested my cheek on the top of her head, and played with that lopsided ponytail.

"Not only because you sign," Bekah told me after the hug.

"Why else?" I asked. Bekah shrugged, "maybe another mom wouldn't bring me here, or . . ." she pointed to her backpack, "let me spend eight dollars for toys for the airplane."

On our way out of town, Bekah took pictures of everything. We have shots of our rented car, the pilot and co-pilot, and several of the kid who sat in front of us on the plane, making faces over the top of his seat. At home, she made a scrapbook from all the photos that we took on our trip.

On the birthdays since our visit to Colorado, Bekah is always delighted to receive Suzanne's gifts and cards—she doesn't cry about missing her any more. She puts the photographs into her album and places the gifts on a special shelf in her room with the handpainted plate. Everything, it seems, is in the right place.

MERRIL MUSHROOM

Jessie's Story

I was stacking firewood when my daughter hollered that our adoption/ foster care caseworker was on the phone. In my haste, I misplaced the next logs and the end of the stack slid down. I was a little annoyed by the time I got inside and on the phone, and I was even more annoyed after I heard why the worker was calling.

"I'm going to try to talk you into taking a child in long-term foster care," she said. "I know you requested to be available only for temporary care in emergencies, but this *is* a kind of emergency. Um, to be perfectly frank, I think you're the only ones who are gonna be able to handle this kid."

Oh great! I thought. And exactly where are we supposed to be able to put this kid? The reason we'd requested to be available only as an emergency, temporary foster placement was that John and I and our four adopted children completely filled up our little house. If we'd had the space for a seventh person to live with us, we'd have applied to adopt again (we'd promised our only daughter a sister some day, maybe even two sisters, so there'd be as many girls as boys in our family).

Our oldest son was thirteen. He had come to live with us when he was ten weeks old. We knew nothing about his background except that he had been left with food and clothing on the steps of the city foundling hospital. He was easy-going and mellow and had severe learning disabilities. Our eleven-year-old son, who had joined us at age one, was high-strung and hypersensitive and also had learning disabilities. Our daughter, now seven, had been a neglected four-month-old when she came to live with us, and our most recent arrival, also seven, was an emotionally disturbed boy who had been with us for the past two years. All the children were of mixed ethnicity.

We all lived in an old one-bedroom farmhouse, and all four children were crammed dormitory-style into half the attic. Our adoption/foster care worker was aware of the space situation, so I knew that if she was asking that we take a child in long-term care, it was probably a critical situation. "Okay," I sighed, "tell me about this child."

I could almost see her smiling triumphantly at the other end of the wire. "He's five years old. He was expelled from kindergarten. He's been neglected, battered and sexually abused. He's going to be placed for adoption eventually, but right now his behavior is so violent that we can't find a family that will keep him. We've just been asked to remove him from his current foster home." She paused, and I heard her take a deep breath before she continued. "We're really hoping you'd consider taking him in a long-term placement. We think you would be able to help him get his behavior under control enough so that he can be placed for adoption. We don't want to have to move him again until he can be adopted."

"How many placements has he been in already?" I asked.

"Four."

Four!! "And how long has he been out of the birth home?"

"Two and a half weeks."

This was sounding worse by the minute. "How long has he been where he is now?"

"Since the day before yesterday."

"My God! What does he do? I mean, the poor kid is only five years old . . ."

"Oh, you know. He's defiant, destructive, uses bad language, spits, kicks . . ."

So far, so good, we'd handled that kind of behavior before. "Does he set fires?" I voiced my greatest fear.

"Not that we know of."

"Well"—I asked about my next area of deep concern—"What kind of preparation has he had for any of these moves? How much follow-up after he has moved? Did he have the changes explained to him?"

"Huh?"

Uh oh. I was afraid of that. This was not a good sign. I sighed again. "Hold on."

I went into the kitchen where John was cooking supper and repeated what the caseworker had said. "It sounded pretty urgent," I finished. "There's not really time to sound the other kids out about this."

"How can we say no?" John responded as I'd anticipated he would, like I myself felt.

I went back to the phone and made the commitment: "Okay, bring him on over."

John and I rushed upstairs to manufacture another space in the house, to create an illusion of privacy for another individual. We cleared out the toy area, moved in a cot and curtained the area with walls made of fancy sheets. No sooner had we finished these preparations when a car pulled up and parked at the bottom of the hill. I looked out to see two adults—a man and a woman, our case worker and the boy's—struggling with a child who had both arms and legs wrapped around the rear bumper of the car. They finally pried him loose and walked up the hill with him between them. When they entered the house, I got my first good look at the boy. My stomach knotted.

He was a tiny, pale-white boy with thin brown hair and huge blue eyes. His face was twisted with fear, hate, fury, despair. I was looking at a rapist-batterer-murderer in larva stage. I immediately was afraid that if I sent him away, did not take him in and give him the benefit of my own expertise and experience in working with disturbed children, my daughter might meet up with him on a dark street someday, or someone else's daughter might, or he would come in their window . . .

"This is Jessie," the male caseworker said.

I watched the boy. He was huddled as far back as he could get on a chair in the farthest corner of the room, knees drawn up close to his body, eyes staring at the floor. "You must be very frightened and angry," I said to him. Huge blue eyes flickered upward, gazed across my face, then back to the floor. "I'd be angry and frightened myself if I was jerked around from one house to another and never knew where I was going," I continued. This time the eyes stayed on my face. "You can stay here now," I said. "I know you have a hard time with some grownups. I can work with children who are angry and frightened and confused. You can stay here for a long time, and no one will move you away without discussing it with you first." The eyes stared at me, then looked back at the floor.

"We fixed a space for you with your own bed," I continued. "Would you like to go see it?" Eyes remained on the floor. I waited. Waited. At last the eyes flickered upward again, and the boy gave a tiny, barely perceptible nod. "Well, come on, then." I stood up and headed toward the stairs, and Jessie slid off his own chair and followed me.

Over the next months, we all worked very, very hard. Jessie indeed did all the things the caseworker had warned us about, plus more, and constantly, too. He had been neglected, beaten, raped and tortured in a family where, according to the reports, violence was an everyday fact of life. He had been jerked around by the people in the system, and he had been given no control over his life or his circumstances. He was defiant, destructive, violent, sexually inappropriate, and he *did* set fires. But little by little, very, very slowly, he began to relax, to trust and to disengage from some of his more trouble-some behaviors. And, little by little, we all began to become very attached to him.

Always we were open with him that we were not a "forever family" for him, that our plan was to work with him and help him learn how to "act right," so that some day he would be adopted by another family where he *would* be able to stay forever.

One day, after Jessie had been with us for about five months, he came into my room. "Mom," he announced. I turned in my chair to attend to him. He came close to my knee, looked into my face and said very seriously, "You know, if you and Dad send me somewhere else to be adopted, I'm gonna be *so bad . . .*" He leaned against my leg.

"You really want to stay here, huh?" I said softly.

He nodded. "I really like it here, Mom. I don't want to go live somewhere else."

A week later, we started adoption proceedings, and shortly after that, with permission from our caseworker, we asked Jessie if he'd like to start using our family name. He said he would. He was excited about the adoption, but he asked me constantly if the police would come and take him back to his birth family. I assured and reassured him that they would not.

Shortly after, Jesse went into a tailspin, fell apart and regressed until his behavior was worse than it had been since he first came to live with us. He had nightmares. He engaged in frantic nesting behaviors. He was violent. He had lots of toileting "accidents."

We were patient. We were reassuring. We asked him what he thought was going on for him, what he thought he needed. We tried everything. We tried anything. We told him we loved him, that he could not change our minds about wanting to adopt him by acting that way. We tried to answer unspoken questions. We told him the police and the social workers all wanted him to live with us. We told him we would not *let* anyone take him away from our family. We tried, in every way we knew, to figure out what was going on for him. Nothing helped. His therapist was at a loss. We were at a loss. His teacher was at a loss. He was, too, even though in the past he had always been unusually insightful and articulate about his feelings. Nothing made any sense. A big piece was missing from this puzzle.

I called our caseworker. I had to find out the details around all his separa-tions and placements. All I knew about his history was that he'd been placed in foster care as an infant and then was returned to his birth home, where he lived with his parents and five siblings until the children were all removed. He'd then gone through the rapid succession of foster placements right before coming to live with us. "How long was he in that first foster home?" I asked. "When and how was he returned to his birth home?" I suspected that therein lay the answers, the key to all this.

"I'm sorry," the caseworker said, "but I can't give you information from his files."

"Listen," I insisted, "this is a crisis! I'm not asking to read his files myself. I'm not asking for names or details or personal stuff. I just need you to pick out information I can have about how long he was in these places and under what circumstances he was removed. Remember everything I've been telling you for the past three weeks about how Jessie's been freaking out? Well, we are in deep trouble! I really need you to look through his files, and tell me what, you think, might have some relevance to this. Please?"

"I'm sorry," she said. "I just can't do that. Our policy, you know . . ."

What I knew was that I desperately needed that information, and I didn't think the policy of the department really was to withhold it. I called the Department of Social Welfare and asked for the assistant commissioner over foster care, explaining what I needed and why.

The next day, my caseworker called. A directive had come down from the state level to give me the information I was requesting. The worker had gone through the files, and what she told me was exactly what I needed to know.

Jessie had been placed in care with the McFoster family at birth. He remained with them for over three years. He was the only child, and the McFosters wanted to adopt him. In spite of the fact they were repeatedly told Jesse was not free for adoption, the McFosters told *him* that they were going to adopt him. They repeatedly sabotaged visits with the birth family and called the toddler Jessie McFoster. Then the McFosters moved out of state and were not permitted to take Jessie with them. He was removed from their home with no preparation or explanation and deposited back with his birth family. At the age of three and a half, he was the third oldest of six children, and because he was a relative stranger, he became the scapegoat in a violent, abusive household.

I could hardly wait to relate this information to Jessie. "Honey," I said, "wait until you hear what I just found out about *you*." In simple language, I told him the series of events. "No wonder you freaked out when we told you we'd adopt you. To you, because of that past experience, being adopted meant going back to your birth family, because that's exactly what happened with the McFosters. But this time, with us, it's different. That won't happen this time. No one will take you back to your birth family anymore. I promise."

"How do you know?" he asked.

"Because this time the caseworkers *want* us to adopt you. They told the

McFosters they *couldn't* adopt you, so the McFosters shouldn't have told you they would. But, the caseworkers told us we *can* adopt you. And we *will*."

Jessie was quiet for a moment. Then he said, "You know, Mom, I had forgotten about all of that, but now I'm beginning to remember . . ." Suddenly fury shone in his eyes. "They had no right to do that to me!" he choked.

"What, Jessie?"

"Those caseworkers, they had no right to do that to me. No one asked *me* if I wanted to leave the McFosters. No one asked *me* if I wanted to move to that mean house. They shouldn't have done that!" I could hear the rage in his voice.

"You're right Jessie," I agreed. "They shouldn't have done it that way, and you have every right to be angry about it."

During the week that followed, Jessie asked me several times a day to tell him that story. I did. Finally, one evening, after my five thousandth repetition (or so it seemed), he turned those big blue eyes on me and said, "Thanks, Mom, I think that was just what I needed to hear about." He hugged me then, and left the room.

And, indeed, the crisis was over.

JUDY ASHKENAZ

Indians

My younger daughter, Johana,* was five and a half when she realized that
she looked different from the rest of us.

It happened one night not long before Christmas, almost eight years ago.
As old as she was, I still sang her to sleep most nights, and I was just about to
settle down with one arm around her and launch into my unvarying bedtime medley, starting with "Go to Bed First, a Golden Purse" and winding
up (depending on how quickly she fell asleep) with either "The Skye Boat
Song" or "All the Pretty Little Horses."

But Johana was not about to go to sleep. Instead, she sat up in bed, stretched
out one smooth brown arm and fixed it with a baleful stare.

"I'm not going to sleep," she told me defiantly, "until my skin turns white."

This came out of the blue, in an immediate sense. Still, I can't say I was
surprised. I'd been waiting for something like this for more than two years,
ever since my husband, David, and I, dizzy with altitude and anticipation,
had first met Johana, a round-faced three-year-old with an institutional bowl
haircut, chasing a skittish little dog around the enormous living room in
Bogotá, Colombia, where, after months of waiting, we had finally arrived to
adopt her.

I was so nervous that August afternoon that everything seemed to be breaking up into dots of light. There was a faint hum behind people's voices, never
mind that they were speaking Spanish. I was holding a large plush lamb with
a bell around its neck, purchased back home in Vermont for this occasion.
"*Mira,*" I kept saying, trying to entice Johana, "*mira el corderito!*" It took

---

* The names Johana and Kate are pseudonyms.

me a little while to notice, through the hum and the pointillist haze, that Rosa (the "directress," as she always signed herself, of the orphanage where Johana had lived since her second birthday), along with everyone else in the room, was calling the lamb *la ovejita*.

Johana herself didn't seem troubled by my linguistic lapse. She climbed into my lap, laying to rest my fears that she'd be hostile or withdrawn. *"Mámi,"* she said, tentatively, and took the lamb and held it against her cheek. Not just then, but a few minutes later, she smiled.

We had left our blond, fair skinned six-year old, Kate—our "bio child," as the adoption literature insisted on describing her, as if she were someone we'd cooked up in a lab—at home in Vermont with her grandparents. Pushing Johana on Avenida Quince in our battered umbrella stroller, in and out of the Foto Una Hora and to the bookstore and the dilapidated playground, we did not attract much attention. David and I, both dark-haired and wearing dark, conservative clothes as we'd been advised, could easily have been well-off *Bogotaños*—the only odd note, ironically, was that we were with such an *Indian-looking* child. The wealthy women who ran the orphanage, the smiling young university students who volunteered there and our hired guide and her family were all fair-skinned and European in features. The maids at the hotel, by contrast, were even darker-complexioned and more Indian-looking than Johana.

Johana, safely strapped into *el coche*, as she dubbed the stroller, wiggled a lot and sang to herself, monotonous little chants she must have learned at the orphanage about getting dressed in the morning or putting away her toys at night. *"Ponga los juguetes,"* she sang energetically, turning around from time to time to blow us kisses: *"Un besito para mi mámi, un besito para mi pápi."* What had they told her, we wondered, what did these words, *mámi*, *pápi,'* mean to her? Did she imagine we were her own parents, her birth parents, come back to get her? Fourteen months is such a long time when you're only three years old. It wasn't likely that Johana consciously remembered anything about her earliest years—how, harboring two different kinds of intestinal parasites, she had developed severe malnutrition; how her father had brought her to the hospital and then had been unable to take her home again, so that when her health returned she had gone to live at the orphanage, with fifty other children.

We had pieced together this history from the sketchy documents that came with the assignment letter, but between Rosa's broken English and our halting Spanish, there were a lot of gaps. We would have years to reflect on those gaps, but right then in Bogotá, eager to get through the red tape and get home and put our little family together, we had more pressing things to think about.

Sometimes, back at the hotel, Johana would withdraw, curled up in a corner, scowling and silent. She didn't actually growl at us, but it felt that way. Eventually, she would fall asleep right there on the carpet, and when she woke up, maybe half an hour later, she'd be cheerful again. My Spanish wasn't sophisticated enough to ask her what was wrong, and I doubt that she could have put it into words. When Johana curled up like that—it happened half a dozen times in the nine days we spent in Bogotá—we kept our distance. And that was the only sign she gave us, right then, of knowing that something was not right, not fair, about her life.

David and I had been well briefed on the particular challenges involved in adopting a foreign-born, non-white, "older" child. After my difficult pregnancy, we had inquired about adoption when Kate was just a few months old. Learning that only a handful of healthy white babies were given up for adoption in Vermont each year, we had begun to think about a child from another country or a child past infancy—or both. But the few articles we found on these subjects discouraged us, not so much by the obstacles they described (the challenge of battling a foreign bureaucracy sounded more appealing than the prospect of another high-risk pregnancy with weeks of enforced bedrest) as by their relentlessly upbeat, Pollyanna tone. Couples, even single people, might adopt not just one or two but half a dozen children, some with severe disabilities. But these adoptive parents did not appear daunted; in photographs, they radiated confidence. "We knew this child was part of God's plan for us," they generally said, in one way or another.

We didn't doubt them, exactly, but neither did we share their confidence in divine guidance, and we were discomfited by an unspoken, apparently blithe assumption at the heart of much of the foreign-adoption literature in the mid-eighties: the notion that the best thing that could possibly happen to a poor, brown-skinned child from an impoverished country would be a new life in a white family in the marvelous land of Burger King and Barbie dolls. Was it even fair, we wondered, to bring such a child to the United States to face a life of prejudice, of being "different"—even from her own family?

We questioned everything—our own motives, the motives of the foreign orphanages and the U.S. agencies and the adoption lawyers. We worried about the possibility of baby-selling and even baby-stealing. The foreign-adoption world, in those days, seemed very much a Christian, mainstream

American one—where did secular, left-leaning types like us fit in?

Then, when Kate was two, we met a couple whose two-year-old daughter had been adopted as an infant in Mexico. Like us, these parents were white and already had one child by birth. More to the point, they did not resemble the saintly couples of the magazine articles. They confronted life much as we did, with the peculiar mixture of idealism and skepticism—the relentless, sometimes too high-minded questioning of received wisdom—that characterizes so many of us who came of age in the sixties. Here were people who had shared our doubts and our questions but had been able to get past them. Encouraged, we renewed our inquiries. And as our first tentative steps led us deeper into the maze of intercountry adoption, we came to terms, finally, with our own undiminished desire to raise a second child. By the time we got the phone call from Bogotá telling us about a "lovely, intelligent" three-year-old girl who had suffered from neglect and malnutrition but was now thriving—a child who needed only "lots of love" and a family of her own—we no longer had any serious doubts about what we were doing.

"How wonderful that she'll be bilingual!" friends exclaimed when they heard our new arrival chattering adorably in Spanish. But Johana had other ideas. "*En inglés!*" she said sternly, warning off the visiting troupe of folk dancers from San Salvador who had made the mistake of paying her compliments (*¡Qué linda! ¡Tan bonita!*) in her native tongue. Just as soon as she had learned enough English to concoct hybrid statements like "Doggie *feo!*" and "*Me quito los* shoes *en mi* house," she was ready to put behind her not only the Spanish language, but also most of the conscious memories that went with it. By Christmas, she was nearly as fluent in English as any of her nursery school classmates, with just a few picturesque grammatical lapses. After that, though she still loved to look through the special album we'd made during and just after our ten days in Bogotá, for a long time Johana did not especially want to talk about Colombia or the orphanage or how she used to speak Spanish. Which was as it should be, we reasoned—you do not bring a child into your family to spend the next fifteen years or so reminding her that she is different.

In Vermont there are very few non-whites, and scarcely any *mestizos*, Latin Americans with Johana's mix of Spanish and Indian ancestry. Johana's skin is a pale yellowish tan in winter, darker in summer; her hair is black with random reddish highlights, straight, thick and glossy. Of course we had *talked* about skin color before that December evening, but always in a matter-of-fact way: Johana is the color of coffee-and-cream, we would say, and Kate is peaches-and-cream. Or, Kate has butterscotch candy eyes, and Johana's are Hershey kisses. On a world map, we showed the girls where our own grandparents were born: Russia, Poland, Lithuania, Hungary. And then we pointed to Spain and, of course, Colombia itself, where Johana's ancestors—her birth parents' ancestors, Spanish and Native American—were born.

We had imagined that being Jewish in small-town Vermont might make it a little easier for us to understand how Johana felt. We know a little bit about what it's like to be different, exotic, the Other. "What kind of a name is 'Ashkenaz,' anyway?" people still ask me. Though we have lived in New England for most of our adult lives, and in Vermont for almost twenty years, to some local people we will always be outsiders: flatlanders, New Yorkers, Jews.

But we also didn't kid ourselves—we knew that racism in the United States is different, at least in degree if not in kind, from all these other types of prejudice. Still, the issue never seemed to come up with Johana, or only in a subtle way, in reverse, so to speak, as when acquaintances seemed a little too eager at first to have their children make play dates with her—the hot new multicultural attraction, live from the Third World. Within a year, though, Johana was thoroughly Americanized, one of the gang, scarcely exotic enough to serve as an example of anything to anybody.

Now, having more or less forgotten this early stage, I had to ask myself: When did Johana learn that the color of your skin is a bigger deal—a *much* bigger deal—than where your grandparents were born, or the color of your eyes or of your hair?

The label "Indian," or even "Native American," as I discovered when Johana started school, remains a loaded one. In kindergarten, the children learned to "sit like Native Americans"—cross-legged, very still, attentive. They learned to "write like Native Americans," picture writing of bear tracks and sunbeams and lightning. Their teacher was no racist but, to the contrary, an intelligent and enlightened woman, who had lived in Latin America herself. All this "Native American" learning was done with great seriousness, great respect: a corrective for years of cultural oversight. Nevertheless, it was a study of Native Americans designed for a classroom full of white children, for the simple reason that there had never been an Indian child in the class before. The only face in that classroom that resembled Johana's was the face of the child on the Bread for the World poster, whose enormous, sad brown eyes, so much like her own, stared out all year from the front of the room: a sub-liminal reproach to the kindergartners, a daily reminder of their own good fortune.

Native Americans, I discovered that year, were different, at least superfi-cially, from the Indians of my own childhood. A kids' movie of that season, a terrible movie full of food fights and toilet jokes, had a plot that revolved around some Native Americans who wanted to save their sacred tribal land from rapacious developers. The Indians won in the end, and an "Indian" notion—"you can't own the earth"—was presented as a moral. Nowadays, especially among children, Native Americans are very much the good guys—serene, ecologically aware, in touch with nature—counterposed to the ac-quisitive whites. Indians, after all, were the original recyclers, they used every part of the animals they killed, they didn't drink fruit juice out of little cardboard boxes and then throw the boxes away in the towering, toxic land-fills that haunt our children's dreams as surely as the atom bomb haunted our own. A big improvement, of course, over the grunting, savage "redskins" of the fifties. But Indians are still exotic, still very much the Other. Native Americans, like the idealized Lakota of *Dances with Wolves*, sit cross-legged, wear the occasional feather in the hair, have arcane initiation rites, live in tepees or longhouses or wigwams, and hold onto idealistic, impractical notions like "you can't own the earth."

Now that I was attuned to "Indians," they seemed to be everywhere. In the supermarket, Johana wanted me to buy a certain brand of bottled water. "You *gotta* buy it," she insisted, lugging the gallon jug over and heaving it into the shopping cart, "'cause it's got a picture of an *Indian* on it, and *I'm* an Indian!" And to prove her point she began circling me, clapping her hand to her mouth in war whoops, "*Wau! Wau! Wau!*" This sort of thing happened often enough that I found myself thinking, whenever I looked at my daugh-ter, about Indians: about how it feels to be somebody else's foreigner. The people Johana met never seemed to mean it badly; they meant, if anything, to be flattering. They were enlightened people, for the most part, with progres-sive views. Who would want to be a boring, white-bread American, after all, with all that imperialism and rapacity on your head? Who wouldn't rather be something else . . . an Indian? I remembered certain college classmates, white Protestants from sheltered backgrounds, who wished they were black, or at least Jewish. They imagined some warm, rich, meaningful world—the gospel church, the family seder—from which they were sorry to be excluded. One girl, a Unitarian, took to wearing a mezuzah on a chain. I wasn't offended, exactly, but I wasn't as pleased as she seemed to expect me to be, either. I was puzzled, and it put a little distance between me and her.

I had that same feeling of distance when acquaintances, admiring Johana's good looks or her progress in English or what they politely referred to as her "marvelous energy level," would suddenly free-associate into odd non sequiturs, recalling a film they had just seen or a speaker they had heard about Guatemala or El Salvador. Johana was too young, of course, to be amused or offended by these leaps. And David and I learned to smile. "Hm," we would say politely. "*That* sounds interesting." And we would cheerfully change the subject.

Johana herself, at five, was a sunny, outgoing child, an enthusiast, a leader. "That one's going to grow up to be President," her kindergarten teacher told me with delight (unwittingly hitting on the one occupation to which Johana, as a naturalized citizen, cannot aspire). Still, every once in a while a little crack would open up in her good humor. Once, Johana and Kate were watching a videotape of *Heidi*, and when Heidi went off all alone to Frankfurt, Johana burst into tears and sobbed out, "*I'm* one of those girls!" (How did she figure *that* out? we wondered, but of course being too young to put it into words is not the same as being too young to know it.) And for quite a while Johana turned sour on the whole "Indian" thing. She didn't want to hear about Indians anymore and she covered up their pictures in storybooks.

Indians, however, seemed to be unavoidable. At Thanksgiving dinner, Johana's four-year-old cousin started to sing a song he'd learned at preschool: "One little, two little, three little Indians." We all looked up, surprised that kids were still learning that song. When he got to the last line, with the obligatory modern nod to feminism ("Ten little Indian *boys and girls*"), his mother looked at Johana and then over at me, with a rueful, what-can-I-do? smile.

I smiled back sympathetically. I don't believe in raising children to be politically correct; I've known too many parents who carefully censor sexist fairy tales and substitute mediation for pitched battles, only to find that their daughters still demand Barbies and their sons turn Legos into pistols, just like everybody else's kids. This cousin's mother is a teacher who introduced peace education into her school during the Reagan years, and I'm sure she has always taught her own kids, as progressive parents do nowadays, that the white settlers grabbed the land from the Native Americans, that the Indians weren't the bad guys.

Johana's cousin went on singing: "Put him in a spaceship and send him to the moo-oon, put him in a spaceship and send him to the moo-oon." And we all laughed a little sheepishly, glad that Johana, who'd been upside down the whole time, trying to perfect the headstand she was learning in gymnastics class, didn't seem to have taken it in at all.

Still, here she was just a few weeks later, holding out her arm. The round Hershey-kiss eyes stared at me accusingly, as if to dismiss in advance any argument I might come up with. "Get real, Mom," the eyes seemed to say.

I was not surprised, but I was almost totally unprepared, so I said the first thing that came into my head—the honest thing: "But if you had white skin," I said, "you wouldn't be our Johana—and *Johana* is the one I love, forever and ever." *Forever and ever*: It's the litany you repeat, over and over, to adopted children, to try to make up for what, on some level, they all know: that somebody once, for whatever reason, *gave them away*.

I looked at Johana while she thought about this—was it a con job or not? In the end, though her skin had not changed color, she relaxed. She curled up in the circle of my arm, and I started to sing, and she fell asleep before I even got to "Go to bed last, nothing but brass."

When Johana first came home with us, she used to sleep with her eyes half open. She talked in her sleep, too, muttering unintelligibly in Spanish and then later on in English. This was the sort of thing we'd read about, so it didn't worry us, though it did present some challenges: You had to tiptoe around the house and talk in whispers, or she would wake up. At some point before the end of the first year, this changed, and she began to sleep more or less the way her sister does—relaxed, arms and legs sprawled: a carefree American girl safe in her own bed in her own home. She began to trust us, as kids are supposed to be able to trust their parents, to keep it that way: to keep her safe.

No one can make that promise, of course, not really, not to any child. But we pretend; we say, "forever and ever." Our birth children, our "biological" offspring, rarely question their security. Adopted kids don't have that luxury; the promise has already been broken, at least once. Lying beside Johana that December night, I understood for the first time what I have had to contemplate a hundred times since: To the extent that Johana allows herself to become one of us, to submerge herself in the family and simply *forget about it*, she also begins to look at herself through our eyes. And then the person she sees is, in some sense, a stranger, the Other—someone different from *us*, the only family she knows. But to the extent that Johana is simply *herself*, she can never be completely *one of us*. This paradox, the living expression of all our original misgivings about foreign adoption, can be, at times, too complicated and painful for a little girl—for anybody—to bear.

Usually, of course, Johana keeps these dark thoughts submerged. But from time to time, and without much warning, they surface, always dragging along with them the same old half-buried anger, the same mistrust. In one of the foreign-adoption stories I read many years ago, one of the few that had the ring of truth, a woman described her daughter, also adopted at the age of three, as "still a little strange" five years later—as not quite knowing "how to act in the feeling areas." Johana is thirteen now, and the same can be said of her. That night many years ago, I could only dimly imagine what lay ahead. I stopped singing and turned off the bedside lamp, and then I lay for a long time with my arm around Johana, not quite ready to disengage myself, to leave my daughter, however safely, all alone in the dark.

SHEILA RULE

Sheila and Sean

I'd always wanted to be a mother when I grew up. Well, I finally grew up at about the age of forty. But by that time I was long-divorced and there was no man in sight looking toward "our" future or gleefully calculating that baby would make three. And I was living rather nomadically as a foreign correspondent, decidedly not a lifestyle conducive to maternity or other ventures grounded in stability.

But the yearning to be a mother fights long and dies hard. It was that yearning as much as anything else that threw me against a wall and blocked my exit until I examined my life. What I saw was a life made up of years of longing to be a mother, a good man's partner, a homemaker, a longing to be tied to routine, stability and responsibility for someone else's well-being.

I'd seemed headed in domesticity's direction in my youth, partly due to society's programming, no doubt, but I think overwhelmingly because of personal passion. Of course, I had another career in mind as well; virtually every black woman I knew worked outside the home as a matter of necessity. And, besides, my mother always drilled in her daughters the following: "Be able to take care of yourself." (Sometimes I think I learned my lesson too well; I became intensely independent and rarely asked for help of any kind.) I decided early on that I would be a writer of some sort and from the age of nine or ten would spend St. Louis's humid, soporific summers writing what I passed off as novels, usually written on compact lined stationery. But invariably, those novels had as their centerpiece a very big, very happy, very loving family. In the eighth grade, home economics was my favorite subject. Even as a journalism major in college, I took a couple of home economics courses and enjoyed them far more than the biology, Italian and Journalism

101 that I was required to sit through.

After college, I married the boy next door; well, actually the boy who lived down the street. Now the fantasies would flower into reality, I figured. Wrong. After only a few years and countless emotional storms, the marriage seemed like just so much debris littering our lives. I moved to New York City—and later to Kenya and England and then back to New York—and lived the life of a single woman. I had somehow lost my way to that state of being called motherhood.

But at forty, in the throes of one hell of a midlife crisis (on second thought, maybe it was an unrelenting wake up call), I found a compass inside myself and got my bearings. I had to face the fact that I had inadvertently stolen a part of me from myself and, in order to reclaim it, I had to become a mother Sure of purpose, I decided to adopt a child.

As I write this, I am about nine months into motherhood and life with Sean. That's my son's name. He's four and a half and, you know, the usual. bright, adorable, funny, affectionate. What else can I say; he's a great kid who is a balm to my soul. I am truly blessed. But I think we were meant to be.

I first laid eyes on him in a photograph I had taken my parents, who were visiting me in New York, to the Association of Black Social Workers' adoption services office to look through books filled with pictures and bios of children available for adoption After I jotted down the ones who appealed to me—I was interested in a son between the ages of two and five—the adoption worker handed me a photo of a beaming little boy who had not yet been entered in the book. Something about him reminded me of my sister, Lynn, when she was little; maybe the way he was hamming it up for the camera. My parents and I agreed that he should be added to my list. As it turned out, the other little boys I'd picked had been featured in the books for some time and had a head start in finding homes. They were already spoken for. Sean was the only one still available.

We first met about a year ago at the adoption agency. I arrived, bearing gifts, after a sleepless night in which my anxiety conjured up a hodgepodge of nightmarish scenarios, including one in which he ran screaming from the room at the sight of me and another that had him staying in the room but standing cowering in a corner and refusing to play with me.

Of course, I didn't know who I was dealing with Sean, dressed in a suit and tie, came bearing joy, acceptance and curiosity. He is a gregarious meeter and greeter, a hi-what's-your name how ya-doin-can we talk kind of guy. We hit it off, even though I don't think he initially had a real notion of just who I was and why I was there I told him I was his new friend and that my name was Sheila; he decided to call me "lady" as in "hey, lady." Now Sean calls me "Mommy," a name often preceded by the words "I love you," especially when he thinks he's in hot water or when it's time for him to call it a night. This thing called motherhood is more wonderful than I ever imagined but at the same time unbelievably H-A-R-D and D-E-M-A-N-D-I-N-G, with lots of exclamation marks and absolutely nothing in lower case. Sometimes I feel inept and just want to cry out, "H-E-L-P!!!!" But then again, one of the best lessons I've learned in this journey is that I can put down some of my be-able-to-take-care-of-yourself spirit. While it's still not that easy to put aside my independence—or to fight my basic shyness—I know that when it comes to Sean, I need to do it. I am, after all, his advocate and when you get right down to it, I'm all that he's got. And so I pick up the phone and call a friend of a friend who's never heard of me but who I've heard has children who benefited from lessons that helped prepare them for kindergarten. Or after trying for nearly an hour to remove a splinter from Sean's finger, I take him to pre-school and ask one of his teachers if she's any good at taking out splinters. I even talk to strangers, reluctantly, at Sean's urging.

"Ask that man what that thing is he's carrying, Mommy."

"You ask him, Sean, if you want to know."

"No, you ask him Mommy."

"Oh, alright, OK. . . . Excuse me, but could you tell us . . ."

And I call on friends to help me out, to babysit, to give me guidance, to lend me an ear or a shoulder.

All the while, I'm continually monitoring my behavior, about as much as I monitor Sean's. At least it seems that way. It feels kind of like standing outside myself and watching me watching Sean. Did I come down too hard on him that time? Could I have said that more softly? Good Lord, Sheila (also known at times as Monster Mommy), where's that deep reservoir of patience that you've always been admired for? Am I letting him watch too much television? What's the big deal; why not let him have pickles for breakfast? Do I really have any idea of what I'm doing? Do I really like children? Would it be easier if there was a Daddy in our lives?

This last question is sometimes the hardest because it is the one over which I have the least control. And also because Sean is truly a man's man. He loves to mix it up with men, truly lights up when one enters a room, seems to react to the authority in their voices with greater haste than to the authority in mine. There are good men in our lives but no constant, everyday presence who can be depended on to help guide Sean in the rituals and ways of manhood. So we do the best we can.

On Saturday afternoons, for example, I usually find myself sitting among other African-American mothers outside a seen-better-days auditorium in Harlem. Inside the hall, our sons and daughters are put through their paces as beginning karate students. Sean doesn't particularly like going—too big an emphasis on discipline for him, I think—but I think we've got to give it a chance. The classes are taught by black men who are trying to cloak our sons in a rich coat of virtues, including love of self and others, respect and honor, strength and compassion.

In some ways, making our way to karate every Saturday is akin to standing watch over Sean in a society that places little value on the lives of black men, one that defines them in terms of pathology rather than promise. As a black parent, I must explore these and other ways of the world that white parents rarely consider.

For black children, it is a disheartening reality that even people who mean no harm will harm them with messages of inferiority or invisibility. It is also true that he will run up against children of his own race who may challenge his blackness, as they view his command of English or his interest in academics (if I'm lucky) as "acting white." The minefield of race and class will be everywhere, just waiting for him to take the wrong path or trip. I must help him cross this minefield without instilling in him paralyzing fear or anger. I must help him develop a strong racial identity and pride, while not alienating him from people of other races.

I wish I could stand guard over Sean everywhere and everyday of his precious life. But I know I cannot. For now, just as I check his little body for scrapes and bruises as a matter of course, I also look in his words, gestures or behavior for bruises of an emotional kind, even those I may have unintentionally inflicted.

As evening stakes its claim and I draw the shade in Sean's room, having honored our daily rituals and put him to bed, I sometimes pause to think about what my life was like before he entered it. I contemplate the hectic parade of humanity on the busy street outside his window and wonder where they are going, these people with blank stares, carefree smiles or knitted-brow scowls, and what awaits them at the end of their journey. I think of how, only a few months earlier, I was among them but am now locked into routine and responsibility that doesn't often allow me to be on the streets past dusk. And then, the falling shade obscures my vision and I turn away. I dim the lights, look at my little boy sleeping, make sure he's still breathing (I can't help it) and walk softly out of his room. A sense of peace gently rocks my heart. I enjoy this child so.

NANCY MAIRS

Ron Her Son

Bye, Grandma," says Chris, who is not quite two, raising his round, wide-eyed face and pouting to meet my lips. "Bye, Grandma," echoes Alex, who suddenly, after a week of spurning all advances, raises his face too for a kiss. Angel is crying as I give her a hug. Ron is characteristically stiff and taciturn in the face of feeling, but he lets me put my arms around him and kiss him, and he even hugs me back a little. Then, in a swirl of arms and legs, a bobbing of heads, they are in their huge, battered station wagon, which must somehow convey them—blankets and bottles, clothes and thermos jugs and trinkets from Mexico and disposable diapers—from here to Texas and then on to Key West. The early morning is greyish and humid, unusual for Tucson in September. I stand on the porch in my nightgown and wave even after they've pulled out of sight.

What has just happened should be that commonplace of American family life, the visit of a son and his wife and their two children to Grandma and Grandpa's house. But it's not. What has just happened is, in many small ways, a miracle.

Ron is not, in fact, my son. Although biologically I am old enough to be his mother, his birth would have put a severe crimp in my high-school style—more, would have been a miracle indeed, since I remained a virgin for several years after Ron was born. Not for seven years after his birth would I actually take on motherhood, and even then people thought me (with some reason) too young. And yet he's more my son than anyone else's. George and I have owned ourselves his parents for longer than anyone else has been willing to do. He may be ours by default, but he is ours. He told me so himself, years ago, in a ragged typewritten note I find now in a file of odd documents that

138

account piecemeal for his life with us:

> To Nancy
> To the one who took me in. Who give me food the one who cared for me
> the one who helped me in my hour of need. Who loved me. Here is to a
> wonder person. On her day, Mother's day. HAPPY MOTHER'S DAY
> Love,
Ron her son

Last comer, eldest child: orphan, waif, bad boy: survivor: son.

George found Ron at the Chazen Institute, a school for emotionally disturbed children where George taught during our first year in Tucson. It was, I imagine, fairly typical of such a place: the children badly housed and fed while the director scooped out as much profit as he could and then split for Chicago. I saw a flow chart of the organization once, in the shape of a pyramid, with the director at the top and the students squeezed in at the bottom, falling off the page. George did not think it a good place for children, and so as often as he could he brought the teenage boys he worked with home. Weekends our house was filled with thieves and muggers, I suppose; one boy, I recall, had put his stepmother through a plate-glass window. He was large for his age. In our house the boys were good-humored, often deferential, and very hungry.

George and I suffer from an adoption complex. Usually we have been able to assuage our urge to shelter homeless creatures by a visit to the local Humane Society, whence we have rescued such members of our household as Freya and Gwydion and Vanessa Bell and Lionel Tigress and Clifford-the-Small-Black-Dog. But occasionally we have found ourselves taking in people for weeks, even months. To a German student who wanted to improve her English we gave room and board in exchange for some help with Anne and Matthew when they were small. One summer a Brown student lived with us while he worked for a political candidate we supported. For a year or so we rented a room to a poor and rather helpless young woman recovering from Hodgkin's disease.

These were all, in a sense, transients, however: people with lives of their own, welcome as sojourners to whatever encouragement and companionship we had to offer until they chose to move elsewhere. At Chazen, we found people without the power—legal, moral, emotional—to make any such choice. They might leave, if anyone were willing to take them (many were wards of the state, which meant that their families, if they had any, were either unwilling or unable to take them), but they'd likely be back, to this place or one like it, until they were old enough to be sent to prison. In light of these realities, we were probably destined, from the moment George started teaching there, to try to rescue at least one of the dozens of children he watched come and go and come.

That one was Ron, but how he came to be Ron and not some other I don't remember. He spent one weekend with us, then another, and another, and gradually a ritual evolved wherein George, who was by now teaching at another school, would drive every Friday afternoon out to Chazen to get him. (The school was located in an area, remote at that time, of the Tucson Mountain foothills, and thus needed no barbed wire. Runaways simply had their shoes taken away. But even faced with acres of rocky ground, cholla and saguaro and prickly pear, rattlesnakes and scorpions, a good many of them went "over the hill.") Friday night, Saturday, Saturday night, Sunday, Ron would spend stretched out in front of the television; often he slept right where he lay, though we had a bed for him in the study. Each Sunday night George would drive him back.

At Christmas that year, 1973 it must have been, he told us he was going home for good. His father hadn't actually said so, but he had sent him a plane ticket, and Ron was sure that once he was home, his father would want him to stay. We had him to our house for an early Christmas before taking him to the airport. I don't recall now just what we gave him—clothes, I think, because he was bursting out of the few articles he owned—but I do remember that after opening his gifts, he disappeared. I found him in the back yard, in the dark, crying softly. "You shouldn't have given me anything," he blurted as I put my arms around him. "I don't have anything for you." "Oh, Ron," I told him, "we don't care. You don't have to give us anything for us to love you." He quieted, but I think now that he didn't believe me. Even after he'd lived with us for a couple of years, he didn't understand why we'd taken him in. "Why do you want me?" he shouted through his tears during one of our rare but agonizing fights. "We love you" was never answer enough. In a life in which survival is based on barter, love can be a pitifully small coin.

Shortly after New Year's the telephone rang. "I'm at the airport," Ron told George. "Can you come get me?" Despite our hopes, George and I were not surprised, although we didn't tell Ron so. What we did tell him was that when he felt ready to leave the Chazen Institute, he was welcome to live with us. We had to tell him that. Clearly his father wasn't about to take him. And the longer he stayed at Chazen, the more dangerous the lessons he learned. He'd been sent there in the first place for truancy, and already while there he'd been busted for shoplifting a carton of cigarettes. Too, because the system of behavior modification used by the school was teaching him that the only real power he had was the power of manipulating the wielders of the system, he spent increasing amounts of his energy gauging what he could or couldn't get away with. He was a shy, sad, abandoned child, grieving for his dead mother, tossed out by his father and his new stepmother, growing steadily more sullen and grim and unattractive. We had no idea whether he could survive with us, but plainly he wasn't likely to survive without us.

He took a long time to say yes. I don't mean moments or days. I mean months. During that time he continued to live with us on weekends. In the summer we took him east with us for several weeks as we visited friends and relations. People were polite, but they obviously considered us more than a little gaga: First we'd moved so far west we'd practically dropped off the edge of the earth, and now we reappeared towing this grubby, gawky figure, with neither impeccable genes nor impeccable jeans, his straight black hair to his shoulders and a gold hoop in one ear, who almost never spoke and never, never smiled. Ron, in turn, was faced with a complicated itinerary among clusters of a large and somewhat bumptious family, none of whom he could see clearly, his glasses having broken just before the trip. Had we been testing his mettle by this ordeal, he'd have passed with colors soaring.

At the end of the summer he came to stay.

And it was awful. Let there be no doubt about that. Lest anyone be tempted to sentimentalize the situation (and many have), to exclaim about our generosity in taking him in or his good fortune in being taken in, I must make clear that much of what followed was painful and maddening and exhausting for all of us. George and I were faced with sole and full responsibility for a troubled fifteen-year-old in whose upbringing we had had no hand, whose values and attitudes were alien to us, whom, all in all, we could love all right but didn't much like. Anne and Matthew, then nine and five, were faced with a jealous big brother who tormented them in ways limited only by his imagination, which luckily wasn't very resourceful. And Ron was faced with an established family, whose rituals and demands were often beyond him, and whose motives for incorporating him remained obscure and baffling.

The first demand that we made of him was that he stop watching television, and it was very nearly a killer. I find the noise of a television unbearably irritating—after a while it drives me to clenched teeth and tears—and I might have been able to survive his weekends silently weeping and gnashing, but I was never going to make it seven days a week. Anyway, like many parents, George and I worry about the effects of television, and so Anne and Matthew had grown up with restrictions on weekday viewing: PBS from four to six o'clock, special shows by petition. Cooperatively, our elderly black-and-white set blew a tube the day Ron moved in, and George was leisurely in replacing it. He took about a month, if I remember correctly. During that time Ron spent most of his hours out of school lying on his back on his bed, staring at the blank ceiling as though to will on it images of Gomer Pyle. The rest of us read books and magazines. Before that month was out, Ron had started to pick up books and magazines too, and although he returned to the television every permissible hour once it was mended, logging hours of *Sesame Street* and *The Electric Company*, which may have given him some much-needed skills, as well as the grisly collection of Saturday-morning cartoons, he usually spent some part of each day reading as well.

Ron's lack of basic skills worried us a good deal. One day as we were driving along Speedway Boulevard, surely one of the most hideously commercial main thoroughfares in the country, we realized that he could not read most of the signs we were passing but was identifying the stores and restaurants by appearance and logos. Neither George nor I had ever known anyone except tiny children who couldn't read, and we were dismayed. A psychologist at Chazen had told us that although Ron's tests revealed average intelligence, his emotional problems would probably keep him from realizing his full abilities. But at least, we thought, he had got to be able to read. Functional literacy took on lively meaning for us. We began to set him tasks we thought would give him survival skills in a literate society. When we traveled, he read the maps and gave directions, and we never got hopelessly lost. We encouraged him to use the bus system, figuring out times and connections. We ate everything he cooked for us except the batch of brownies for which he misread one-half teaspoon as one-half cup of baking soda; those heaved and crawled up the sides of the pan and all over the oven and were thereby lost to us.

Ron's schooling helped some, of course. We sent him to the Catholic high school of not quite a thousand students where George and I were teaching, in the hope that the atmosphere there would be less daunting than that at the public high school, about three times Salpointe's size, to which he would have been assigned. He had, after all, been incarcerated for truancy, and school obviously held for him terrors that we didn't know but certainly believed. In his two years at Salpointe, he missed two half-days, both with my permission. And although his ability to read and write and figure was still marginal when he graduated, it was at least sufficient to satisfy the Navy.

In many ways, Ron's lack of social skills was more troubling than his lack of academic skills. He had no idea how to form and sustain relationships either within the family or without. Over time, as we began to piece together from various sources the details of his history, we began to understand why he was able neither to give nor to receive the ordinary gestures of human warmth and attachment. What we learned took us well beyond our experiential and conceptual boundaries.

According to a letter from a woman, located by our lawyer as she tried to trace Ron's origins to satisfy guardianship requirements, little "Roddy" was born on 1 October 1958 in Fort Yukon, Alaska, the illegitimate child of an American soldier and an Athabaskan woman. The Athabaskan woman, married with several children already, took him home, but after about a year the tribe told her that she could no longer keep him because he was too white. She took him, hungry and covered with sores, to the woman, who agreed to keep him; but when he was about four, she and her husband divorced. She then gave him to friends who had no children of their own. How accurate this information is we don't know, since we have copies of both a baptismal certificate from St. Stephen's Episcopal Church in Fort Yukon for Elwood Roderick Gabriel, dated 23 November 1958, and a certificate of live birth, dated 3 October 1958, of Elwood Roderick Rose.

At any rate, the couple took him in and renamed him Ronald William DuGay, according to a copy of a baptismal certificate dated 3 July 1962. They raised him, and eventually the man legally adopted him, though not until 8 November 1973. Some time before, his wife had died of some neurological disease. Within six months, he had remarried, a woman with a teenage son of her own, who wanted nothing to do with Ron; and so Ron was made a ward of the state of Colorado and sent to Chazen (whose stiff fees were paid for by the federal government since the man was an Army veteran) for refusing to go to school. While Ron was there, we discovered in the elaborate course of obtaining guardianship, which required the man's permission, he moved from Colorado to California without leaving a forwarding address. The sum of these events was a sharp message: Don't settle in too deep, don't put out tendrils of affection: The tendrils will be hacked away: Whoever you love will leave you. I have said that Ron had some learning difficulties, but he was not stupid. He learned this lesson by heart.

Our relationship with Ron's father, whom we never met, was complicated and bitter. I had forgotten, in fact, just how painful it was until I dug out Ron's file and old furies flew out of the folder and gripped me in talons amazingly sharp for all their age. Once we had tracked him down, the man was glad enough to sign the guardianship papers, a legal necessity in case Ron ever needed emergency medical care. Indeed, clearly he wanted to be quit of Ron altogether. He refused to support Ron, or even to send him the few possessions—a bicycle, a Boy Scout backpack and mess kit, an old pony bridle —that Ron had laid up. To get these I used, in one of the ugliest machinations of my life, the only leverage I knew I had: "Unless Ron's things are in his possession by Thanksgiving," I wrote him, "we will return Ron to you. If you will not *share* the responsibility for your son with us, then you must assume *full* responsibility for him." They arrived by Greyhound within a week.

The issue of support was not so readily resolved. Both teachers, George and I made too little money to enable us to take on another mouth to feed, another frame to clothe, especially one that ate and grew prodigiously. But because the man was not an Arizona resident, we could not be paid foster parents under the Arizona Department of Economic Security. The authorities in California rejected a reciprocal agreement, though they would have supported Ron in a foster home in their own state. Our point was not just to get Ron foster care, however; it was to care for him in our own family. At one point the man agreed to send us twenty-two dollars a month, but after two months the checks stopped. Finally, the Veterans Administration arranged garnishment of twenty-five dollars a month from his retirement check, and we had to make do with that. Ron always had enough to eat, I think, but he had few clothes, and with five dollars a week for allowance he could afford few indulgences.

Ron's father may not have been very much to blame in his negligence. He was, according to one of his daughters by his first marriage, a "weak" man who had to have a woman to lean on, and so she was not surprised that he remarried precipitously without caring whether his new wife and Ron could get along. Anyway, I think Ron had been pretty much his mother's child, and she was dead. The man's intelligence and education seemed limited, and he certainly knew nothing of child psychology: It seemed never to have occurred to him that Ron's behavior was connected to what was going on in his life. Too, he was aging, with a heart condition; all he wanted was peace and ease. And Ron, smoldering with grief, resentment, rage, was a difficult and threatening presence. I know. I lived with him.

The people who suffered most immediately from that presence were Anne and Matthew. Ron resented them, of course: They were the "real" children, whose places in the family could never be doubted, whereas he was among us by sufferance, in a position more tenuous in his perception than in actuality. We did not want to get rid of him, but nothing in his experience had taught him that human ties could be so tenacious. I think he always lived on the edge of expulsion. Nothing had taught him gentleness either. The only words he knew to reach the children were threat—"I'm gonna break your arm"—and the only touch a swat, a pinch, the quick wrench of a limb, the yank at a lock of hair. One night he so menaced Matthew that

Matthew, in flight, smashed one arm through a glass door, severing the ulnar artery and two tendons.

We were asking a lot of two quite young children. Today I wonder whether we asked too much. The scar on Matthew's wrist is, after seven years, a thin silvery thread. But are there other scars, I wonder, elsewhere than in the flesh, puckers in mind, in emotions, from those years of living with an almost aimless meanness? When I ask the children their feelings about the time Ron lived with us, Matthew's memories are fond, Anne's bitter. Matthew is glad Ron was there, he says—Ron was "fun." Anne makes the kind of face I have learned to associate with her refusal to express strong anger openly. "Do you wish he hadn't come to live with us?" I ask. "I was so young," Matthew explains, "that it never occurred to me that Ron wasn't just part of the family." "And I," says Anne, "was used to beating up on Matthew but not to getting beaten up on myself." We laugh at this discovery of different perceptions according to place in the family. Matthew, at the bottom of the pecking order anyway, seems to have figured that Ron's bullying was just part of family life; for Anne he shifted the entire familial structure. She punished him cruelly for his intrusion, though she looks surprised now when I tell her so. Far brighter and more self-assured than he, she outwitted him at turn after turn, jeered at his mistakes in reading, pronunciation, and simple math, lashed him verbally. Many of his pinches and slaps may have been retaliatory, as a bear swats at the bees that sting his ears and nose when he raids their honey. Matthew, with the lovely warmth he has had since he was a toddler, overwhelmed him in quite another way: He forgave Ron every blow, every trick, and loved him relentlessly, mean spirit and all.

From Ron's point of view, life in our family must have been a sore trial. We were told by his counselor at Chazen that he needed a firmly structured environment, but even without such a caution, the need would have been clear. He was the most passive child I have ever known—emotionally, intellectually, even physically inert. When he stood and walked, his small bony frame seemed to be melting; whenever he could, he lay limply on his bed or in a chair. He could not think of things to do, even to amuse himself; he lay still for hours, as though waiting for something to happen to him. He rarely laughed, and then—a quick bark—only if someone were hurt or humiliated in some way. Nor did he cry as a rule, or complain, or rebel. He was the only student George had known at Chazen who never once tried to run away. He was unnervingly tractable. He would do whatever one demanded. Of course he would do it as quickly and badly as he could get away with, but so will most children; his carelessness was, in an odd way, a healthy sign. His pliancy was scary. The firm structure we were advised to give him seemed necessary literally to give him a form, keep him intact, so that he wouldn't dissolve and ooze away.

And so we were strict in our requirements and regulations. Ron had to attend school every day and a counseling session once a week. He had to do enough work in his classes to enable him to pass. His fixed household chores were to wash the dishes and to keep his room decent, though not necessarily spotless; in addition, we expected him to pitch in for routine cleaning, shopping and yard work. If he went out, as he too seldom did, he had to tell us where he was going and when he'd be back. Phone calls were limited to fifteen minutes, though often, after he'd begun to make friends, he trotted to the nearest pay phone and chatted to his adolescent heart's content. He was not to drink alcohol, smoke dope or take anything that didn't belong to him; on these points we were adamant, knowing that, with his record, he could be whisked at the slightest infraction into the juvenile-detention system and we would be helpless to keep him. Anne and Matthew must meet a nearly identical set of demands now that they are teenagers—we didn't create them especially for Ron—but Anne and Matthew have grown up with our expectations, under our discipline. For Ron, adapting to them, suddenly and wholesale, must have been a harsh and often bewildering task.

Living closely with him, we could not always tell whether Ron was making progress. But gradually he was. His first quarter at Salpointe he was enrolled in the physical education course required for graduation. He had, it turned out, some sort of hang-up about P.E., the nature of which we never discovered, though we gathered that it was partly responsible for his earlier truancy. At mid-quarter we received notice that Ron was failing P.E. because he had never attended. Confronted with the failure warning, he acknowledged that he had just gone off and sat under a tree every day during first period.

"What did you think would happen when we found out?" we asked him.

"I thought I'd get to the mail first," he said.

"But we'd still have found out at the end of the quarter."

Ron seemed nonplussed. He probably hadn't thought that far ahead. He was even more nonplussed when we told him he'd simply have to take P.E. another time. Evidently he believed that by his failure he'd cleared himself of the obligation somehow. Quarter after quarter he put it off, waiting, I suppose, for some sign of our relenting. In the last quarter of his senior year, dressing out with a flock of freshmen and sophomores, he took P.E. and passed it. He passed all his other courses as well, though perhaps he shouldn't have. We refused to teach him ourselves, but his teachers were our friends in this small, intimate faculty, and they may have been more kind than honest. He made a few friends and began to wander off campus at lunch to sneak cigarettes and "fool around." He even got hauled into the dean's office one day for getting into a fight. Our bony lump, who had never dared take on anything bigger than a ten-year-old girl, lashed out at another boy just before religion class. We could not condone the act, but we rejoiced in the energy behind it.

As Ron's senior year waned, we grew increasingly worried about his future. Clearly he was going to graduate, with only marginal skills and even poorer initiative. He didn't seem capable of college-level work, even at our local community college. And although one of our demands when he came to live with us had been that he get a part-time job, he had never done so; he claimed to have tried, but we doubted that he had ever screwed his courage so far as to request and fill out an application. He seemed an unlikely candidate for success in the tightening job market. But we would not keep him, we were sure. We were still financially distressed: Anne was old enough to need a room of her own instead of sharing one with Matthew; most of all, we were exhausted. At least by the time he was eighteen, Ron would have to go off on his own.

We were rescued in the most ironic way possible. Ron was incapable of independent action, but he would do as he was told. He needed, then, a situation in which every aspect of his life and work would be regulated. Holy orders offered one alternative, but on the basis of his overweening interest in girls, he did not seem in the least cut out to be a priest. The second most paternalistic organization we could think of after the Catholic church was the military. Two pacifists, radicalized by the grinding ugliness of Vietnam, George and I found ourselves recruiting our foster son for Uncle Sam. His father had been in the Army, of course, and Ron would not, even fleetingly, consider enlistment in the same branch of the service; by this time his fury at his betrayal by his father was flinty. But George had been a naval officer for three years in the early sixties, and George was apparently—though Ron could probably not have said so—okay. Ron took himself to the Naval Recruitment Office, passed the tests, signed the papers. We were all free.

Or almost. We had tried to teach Ron to be scrupulous. Soon after he came to live with us, while we were waiting in line one day at McDonald's, Ron showed me a pair of sunglasses he had lifted from a nearby Circle K. Why is it that children choose to administer these tests in the agora, while you are trying to order three Big Macs and two Quarter Pounders, two Cokes, a Dr. Pepper, a root beer, and a Sprite, and No thank you, you wouldn't like some hot apple turnovers for dessert with walls of polyestered shoulders on every side and your five-year-old unloading an entire napkin-holder just beyond your clutching fingers? I told Ron quietly but, I hoped, emphatically that he was not to take things that didn't belong to him, because shoplifting was against the law and we would lose him if he were caught, and that he was to return the sunglasses to the Circle K. I don't know whether he did, but I never saw them again. Nor did I see evidence of other booty, though he was painfully poor compared to most of his classmates and may have succumbed to temptation, especially with regard to a turquoise ring I had given to George which disappeared without a trace.

We were equally strict about truthfulness, and I remember Ron blazing with anger once when I lied to the telephone company, telling them I didn't have an illicit extension phone, to save myself some embarrassment. He accused me of being no better than he had been when he tried to cover up his failure in P.E.; and he was right. How often our children keep us honest. So it was not surprising that, when the Navy recruiter asked him whether he had ever smoked marijuana he said that he had. There was a six-month waiting period after the last incident, he was told, and so he could not go into the Navy in August as planned but would have to wait till October.

I nearly wept when I heard of the delay. I was tired—I had just finished a difficult school year, I had not been rehired, the summer heat that aggravates multiple sclerosis symptoms was in full force—and one of the things I was tired of was Ron's presence, especially his ceaseless bickering with the children. And now I was faced with two extra months of it. But as I look back, I'm glad he had the extra time. He still claimed that he couldn't find a job, but once he had graduated I was no longer willing to let the matter slide. He was now, I told him, an adult, and adults had to assume responsibility in society; if he couldn't find a paid job he'd have to do volunteer work. So he spent several months at the Red Cross, lugging bags of blood about twenty hours each week, and the people there seemed to think well of him. He needed that success. Also, Anne had been promised her own room for her eleventh birthday in September; rather than renege, we simply moved Ron in with Matthew, freeing his room to be redecorated for Anne. Ron was rather nice about his own space and possessions, and I think he began to be eager to escape Matthew's miasma. By the end of the summer, too, his friends had drifted away, into college or jobs. Without the familiar structure of high school, without his own room, without old friends or any way to make new ones, he could look forward to the Navy with some enthusiasm.

Shortly after his eighteenth birthday, we put Ron on a Greyhound for basic training in San Diego, a skinny, slouching, silent young man with shaggy dark hair and dark-framed glasses, wearing jeans and an open-necked shirt, though as I recall the earring was gone. I don't know whether he was terrified, but I know that I was. He was, after all, my eldest child, the first one to go off, and he seemed more fragile and vulnerable than either of the others. George and I had tried to make the world solid for him and to give him some of the skills we thought he'd need to survive, but we'd had so little time, and we'd made so many mistakes: Most parents get eighteen years; we'd had, all told, not much more than three. I watched the bus pull out of the station and down the narrow street, and when I couldn't see it anymore, I watched the point at which it had disappeared, as though I could fix myself to it somehow and travel with Ron across the desert, over the rubbly mountains, down to the blue sweep of San Diego Harbor, where once, on a vacation, we had all gone onto the base and stood under the looming grey ships.

The first separation was short, for Ron was allowed to come home at Christmas. At the airport we couldn't find him; he had to find us. Who was this man in the shirt and tie, the dark uniform and white cap, black stubble covering his round pink head, almost smiling as we reached out to pull him close, almost hugging us back? He was our Ron, and he wasn't. Already he was different. Quiet, not sullen, but quiet, at ease. He teased the children, not as one child taunting others but as a big brother showing off a bit. He brought us fine presents—I still keep my jewelry in the handsome white case with the red satin lining. He talked to us. And then suddenly he was gone again.

We saw him only once more, the following fall, when he had finished radio school and was on his way to a ship in Norfolk. In May 1978 he called to tell us he'd just gotten married to a girl called Angel. In June 1979 his first son was born: Alexander William Randall DuGay. In August 1980, about to be transferred to Keflavik, Iceland, the three got as far as Waco, Texas, to visit Angel's mother, but they couldn't afford the trip to Tucson and we couldn't afford the trip to Waco. In Keflavik, in October 1980, Christopher Jason Allen DuGay was born. Now George and I had a daughter-in-law and two grandbabies we'd never seen. And then at last this summer, between Keflavik and their new duty station in Key West, they came to us.

How strange to see Ron with his wife and children. In five years he has changed some—filled out, grown self-assured—though not so drastically as he did during that first brief separation. Angel I have come to know and like through her good letters. She is the kind of person I enjoy: alert, thoughtful, an enthusiastic tourist, who loves to read and keeps a journal. I worry about her a good deal because, like me, she is easily depressed, and I think that her life, with two such small children, is difficult just now; but so far her courage hasn't failed. At least while he's on leave, Ron takes turns with her watching the boys, who need surprisingly little watching; I've tried to childproof the house, putting our few fragile treasures out of reach, and the only thing that seems in any danger is Lionel Tigress, the new kitten, whom they plaster with pats and sticky kisses. Ron's involvement seems natural, genuine. Almost immediately the night they arrived, Alex threw up all over the dining room, and while Angel raced him to the bathroom, Ron grabbed a roll of paper towels and started mopping. I know a good many men who'd have sat frozen waiting for some woman—and although Angel was otherwise occupied, Anne and I were both available for duty—to cope with the mess. I liked him a lot then. I liked his calm, his competence.

They act like a family. They are a family. Ron has for the first time in his conscious life his own kin, people whose relationship is clear and unequivocal, who belong to him, to whom he belongs, not by sufferance but by right. And he has brought them home to us—home, here, where we are—because we are part of the family, eight of us under one roof. I sense that he has owned us—really owned us, with that matter-of-fact boldness with which children recognize their parents and their siblings—at last. Us: Grandma, Grandpa, Aunt Anne, Uncle Matthew, to whom Alex and Chris, through their father, now have every claim.

People have asked me often whether I regret taking Ron in, whether I'd do so again if I had it to do over. Hard questions to face, the answers risky to the ways I like to think of myself.

Because I did regret taking him in, many times. I lack the largeness of spirit that enables someone like George to transcend daily inconveniences, lapses in behavior, even alien values, and to cherish a person without condition. I often judged Ron harshly, by standards inappropriate to his peculiar situation; I was often grudging of approval and affection; I made him work too hard for the privilege of being my son. He suffered, I'm afraid, for my regrets. And no, I think, I wouldn't do it again, knowing what I now know. But then, I wouldn't have Anne and Matthew again either. Might not even marry George again. Such ventures seem now, in the wisdom of hindsight, to demand a woman of more than my mettle. That's how we get wise, by taking on in ignorance the tasks we would never later dare to do.

No. Yes.

ADOPTED DAUGHTERS

ME-K ANDO

Living in Half Tones

Recognition. Likeness. Familiarity. Most people take these things for granted. They look at themselves, and then at their parents. They try to find the likeness, the similarity, and most of the time they are successful: They can see where their nose came from; the curl of their hair; the thickness of their waist. They know who conceived them. There is never a question.

I have never felt that recognition, that certainty. People look at me, and don't know what to think. They see my Asian features and my mother's Asian features and assume she is my birth mother. They look at my white father and they are confused. How could this white man and this Asian woman have conceived me?

"Where were you born?" they ask.

"In Korea."

"Isn't your mother Japanese?"

"Yes . . . Okay. Okay. I was adopted from Korea. My third mother is Japanese, and my father is Swedish and German. I'm not Japanese, and I'm not white. I'm Korean. My brother is also Korean. And adopted. We have a unique family."

People look at me in bewilderment. I don't know how many actually understand my explanation. My third given name, which I used until this past year, was in itself hard enough for them to figure out: Karen Hiroko Muckenhirn. American Japanese German. None of which I am. It is all a reconstruction. Somebody else defining who I was and who I would become. A manufactured identity. My second given name is Baik Me Kyung. *Baik* is

Korean for white. White after my second mother, June White, the American woman who took me into her orphanage. *Me Kyung* because it was a "pretty" name. I still don't know what my first given name was. I don't know if I had a name.

I grew up thinking that I was more Japanese than Korean. Korea, that mysterious hidden space in the sky of my past, was my known birthplace, but I saw *my* eyes in my Japanese mother's eyes. For years, I hated them. They represented the pain and suffering in my life. So I would gaze into my father's big light blue eyes and get lost in them. And I would stare at my friends' blue eyes and envy them.

I thought my third parents were my only parents. The orphanage in Chechon, Korea, was nothing but a dot hidden, shielded from my earliest memories. My mother was my mother, and my father, my father. There was no one else. For years, I looked at my mother but didn't really see her. I could only see my father's pale white skin, light blue eyes, light-brown hair. He represented what I was supposed to become.

I know now that my third parents weren't my only parents. I know that June White was my second mother. I still don't know who my birth mother was. Over the past three years, I have seen my Japanese mother more and more—I mean really seen her. I feel lucky to have been adopted by at least one parent of Asian descent. I can't imagine having two white parents.

Sometimes I feel my life would be different if I just knew what my birth mother and father looked like. I want to be able to see my eyes in my first mother's eyes, to know where the shape of my legs came from, the softness of my nose, the paleness of my skin. If I could just see a photograph, maybe all these years of feeling displaced and disconnected could be transformed.

My journey to find my first mother's eyes began last August when, at twenty-five, I returned to Korea for the first time. It was there that I met my second mother, and it was there that the purpose of my journey became clear.

"May I have your attention please," a voice screeched over the loudspeaker. "We will now begin general boarding for Northwest's Flight 303 to Kimpo International Airport in Seoul, Korea. Please have your boarding passes ready. Thank you."

My mother and I slowly rose from our seats in the waiting area. We had arrived at the Seattle airport from Minneapolis more than three hours earlier. As we boarded the Boeing 747 for the ten-hour flight, I wanted to escape into a shelter of sleep. Being trapped in a plane with only the Pacific below was too much to think about.

I pushed my seat back as far as it could go, fumbled with my seatbelt and then reached to grab the small pillow with the white, gauze-like covering. As I leaned over a worn yellowed photograph fell out of my jacket pocket. It was a photo of June White, the director of the orphanage. The picture had been taken years ago, supposedly at a gathering where I originally met her. I had no recollection of it. She was still in Korea twenty-three years after my departure.

I wrote to her on two occasions. After the first, I received no reply. The address was given to me by the adoption agency, so I assumed that it was accurate. Maybe she was no longer there. Maybe the orphanage no longer existed. The unanswered letter came as no surprise. Three months later I received a phone call.

"Is Karen there?" a woman's voice asked.

"This is she."

"My name is Gail Karlin. I received a call from your father that you wrote to June White in Korea about your plans to travel there soon," she said.

"My dad called you?" I asked her. "When was that?"

"Oh, it was last week sometime. He asked me to call you."

My dad had this way of surprising me at certain important times in my life. Our sporadic communication lacked the ease I expected between father and daughter. We never talked about adoption.

"Um, yeah. My mom and I wanted to take a trip there sometime in August or September. Who are you?"

"Oh, I'm sorry. I'm June's assistant here in Minnesota. I take care of her correspondence in the States."

"How did my dad make contact with you?"

"He probably called the agency first and they probably referred him to me. Anyway, how are you doing?"

"Uh, I'm all right." I didn't understand her familiar demeanor.

"How is your mom? She's Japanese, right?"

"Did my dad tell you? How did you know?"

"I just remember your family. I've been working with June for quite a while. I met your parents on a couple of occasions."

"Really?" I wondered why my parents had never told me about her. She lived so close, and she probably had a lot of important information. Were they trying to hide something from me?

My feelings about adoption had been ambivalent up until this point. I knew that I had been born in Korea, that I had lived there for the first two years of my life, but Korea was merely a name to me; a place that, for one reason or another, had told me "We cannot take care of you." It was a place where I did not belong. Until recently I had never envisioned actually returning, let alone looking at any of my records. I was still trying to figure out what being adopted meant. It was scary to think about. Talking to Gail forced me to think about it more concretely. We had three more months.

Gail called me one month later to tell me June had finally received my letter. June had called her the night before, and they had talked about my future visit.

"Will we be able to stay with her, or should we get hotel accommodations?" I asked.

"Oh, no, no, she has a really big place. There's plenty of room. You're more than welcome to stay there."

As she talked, a picture of the orphanage slowly began to take shape in my imagination. It was a two-story Victorian style house. White. Old. Rundown. It needed a paint job. Not too far away was a tiny playground. A couple of wooden swings. A seesaw.

"Oh, she also mentioned the possibility of meeting you at the airport. Once in a while, she takes some of the kids up to Seoul for their physicals. So, if she is up there on that day, she can pick you up."

My heart fluttered. I was both excited and scared at the same time. Until now, I thought that we would have to make our own way down to Chechon. That June wanted to meet us at the airport made me think that she really did care about me. Maybe she even remembered me. More and more, the eerie reality of my return sank in.

Two weeks before we left, Gail called to say that June would be at the airport.

As I lay back on the cramped airline seat, I began to think about what our meeting would be like. June would now be a part of welcoming me back to my homeland. I imagined that she would recognize me after all these years and run toward me, excited, arms outstretched. She would reconnect me to Korea. Knowing exactly what I was going through on this first visit back, she would make me feel special. Her enthusiasm and emotional reaction would disarm my inhibitions, and I would feel wholly bonded to her, my "second mother." I dreamed that when the airplane arrived in Korea, I would feel as though I had returned home: that I would experience a spiritual connection as the American plane's wheels made contact with Korean soil.

When the plane began its descent and the scattered landscape of Korea took shape, I struggled to breathe. The realization that I was returning was slow, intense. It was like trudging up a steep mountain toward the thin new air offered at the peak. My mother was nervous, her head bobbing up and down in short, quick movements. She kept telling me on the plane, "You shouldn't expect too much. Don't get your hopes high, you'll just get disappointed." Her expression was sad, worried and concerned at the same time.

I just shook my head. "Mom, I've told you. I know I shouldn't expect anything." I was tired of her advice. "I have no idea what's going to happen. How could I be disappointed? This is going to be an exciting trip," I said trying to hide my uncertainty.

I walked through the crowded receiving line in the expansive airport lobby clutching June's photo. My mother followed me. I didn't want to look back at her: I only wanted to find June. Gail had told me, "Look for a lady with light-reddish hair. She'll be tall, and she wears glasses." I thought it would be obvious. I had heard that Korea was one of the most homogeneous countries in the world, but many Caucasians were on the plane bound for their military posts. As I walked past the last person in the line, I twisted around slowly, looking back through all the Korean faces I had passed. Maybe something had happened. Maybe I had missed her in my anxious confusion.

I stood for a while and scanned the lobby. A tall woman wearing a navy, cotton A-line skirt and a matching striped shirt appeared and then disappeared behind a large group of bodies complete with name tags and identical luggage. Must be a tour group, I thought.

I headed toward the group, hands clenched. The striped shirt appeared again. I felt the sweat forming on my forehead. I stopped and looked around for my mom. Waiting by a pillar with our luggage, she gave me a concerned look with her weary eyes. The ten-hour plane ride had taken its toll. I turned around and briskly walked towards the stripes.

"Uh, are you June?" I asked. My voice was thin, barely audible.

"What?" she asked.

I cleared my throat and tried again. "Are you June White?"

"Yes," she said flatly. The expression on her face did not change. Her hands remained tightly wrapped around her white vinyl purse.

"I'm Karen," I said, trying to smile. I extended my hand toward her, but I quickly pulled it back when she began to talk.

"We saw you walk into the line, and we tried to signal you, but you didn't see us," she told me, pointing toward the entrance of the lobby. She looked nervously at her assistant, Mrs. Kim, who had made the long journey with her. She said something to her in Korean and looked at me again.

I shifted back and forth from foot to foot, staring at Mrs. Kim and then at June. Mrs. Kim looked at me and then whispered to June. I searched for something to say. I felt as though I were sinking in my own fabricated reality.

My mom tapped me on my shoulder, breaking the awkward silence.

"Mom, this is June."

"Oh, yes, yes . . . I kind of recognize you," she said reaching out toward June's hands. As my mom clenched her short, thick fingers around June's unexpecting hands, it was as if she squeezed all the life out of them. June's large hands just went limp. I looked up at June's face, examining her eyes. She caught my glance, shifted her head back toward my mom and then stared at the beige tile floor.

My mom made small talk. I don't know what she said. My mind was reeling, my eyes watering. I wanted to disappear and start all over again. Maybe this *wasn't* really June. She was too business like. I felt as if I were on an assembly line, another adoptee returning to Korea in search of her scattered missing pieces. I had arrived and then I would leave, just as all the others who had chosen to make this trip into their mysterious past.

"I think we should get going now. It's a long ride back," June said as she turned to leave.

Tropical trees lined the large parking lot full of Daewoos, Hyundais, the cars miniature models of those exported to the United States. Strange hollow sounds bounced against the distant mountain range in a cacophonous roar—car horns blaring, trucks shrieking down the freeway, heavy construction equipment bruising the landscape. It was a bright, sunny day in Seoul, the air so thick it stuck to my skin. I inhaled deeply, following my breath, trying to absorb everything around me.

A few years ago I had mentioned to a friend that sometimes I didn't feel as if I were who I was, as though there were another me inside of me, controlling my mind, separating it from my body. It was as if I were looking out of someone else's eyes. He asked me if I felt this way because I was adopted. He wondered whether my disconnection from my birth parents was related to these feelings.

As I walked up the dark stairwell of the orphanage, I wondered whether those sensations would ever subside. Somewhere in the faraway reaches of my psyche, I hoped that I would remember something about my early life in this orphanage; some memory that would help me shed some light on this other "me." Maybe it would be the bricks in the building. Or maybe something as minuscule as a creak in the floorboards, a scent in the air. But even in the stairwell I could tell that remembering would be difficult. This three-story brick building was so foreign; the difference between it and the shabby white Victorian house I had envisioned was unsettling.

As we walked by the second floor, I spotted several tiny shoes outside the entrance. This must be where all the kids are, I thought. My heart fluttered deliriously. I thought about my crumbling Korean shoe back home, the one treasured item that had survived my journey to the States as a two-year-old. My other shoe had mysteriously disappeared, along with my early past.

Early the next day we climbed up to the top floor to tour the orphanage kitchen and dining room. Suddenly I heard the cries and yelps of children let loose. I rushed out onto the third-floor balcony which overlooked a large playground, my mother following close behind. Peering over the railing, I saw a swarm of tiny black heads scurrying here and there. Loud, high-pitched music blared. The catchy rhythms and melodies were soothing, perhaps to control the children's sometimes erratic behavior. It all looked like an orchestrated flurry of motion.

The children had just been released from devotionals. Not a minute passed before one of the kids spotted us staring down at them. She began screaming something in Korean and several other kids gathered around her, pointing their fingers in our direction. They were all smiling and jumping up and down and running around in circles. Their excitement increased with the soaring midday temperature. Some of them were trying to talk to us. All I could make out was, "Yo, yo!" I looked over at my mom. Her face was full of joy.

"It looks like they want us to go down there!" I exclaimed. I couldn't hide my enthusiasm. My heart began to beat faster. I couldn't wait to join them. Their cries of joy broke my heart.

"Come on, Ma, let's go!" I said, not waiting for a response.

"Okay," she replied, as I whipped by her.

I ran down the three flights of concrete steps. By the time I reached the last set of stairs, more of the kids had gathered at the threshold of the playground. I slowed my pace, scanning all the faces staring up at me. They were all so small, fragile. While I walked toward them, the girl who had first noticed us, ran up and grabbed my hand. She looked up at me, grinning widely, and pulled me toward the others. Her slight body was smaller than most of the others and she wore a short-sleeved red T-shirt with purple shorts. Her thin hair was chin length with short-cropped bangs. Every two or three steps she would glance back up at me and her face would collapse into a sad smile.

As we passed through the crowd of kids, a chubby boy with a stained shirt began tugging at my white top. I looked back at his fat cheeks and smiled. His sad expression forced me to stop. He stared at me and lifted both his arms. He whined something in Korean and started jumping up and down in his tiny sandals. I leaned down and scooped him up. Instantly, he clung to me with such ferocity it startled me. I began to realize how starved these kids were for attention. During my short stay, I wanted to do everything I could to satisfy their hunger.

The chubby two-year-old weighed heavy in my thin arms. It's time to put you down, I thought. But the moment I began to lower him, he wriggled in desperation, clinging to me even closer. I kneeled down with him and let go of his waist. His arms were still tightly wrapped around my neck. I reached behind my head and pried them open. As I pushed him away, I quickly stood up but he immediately grabbed onto my right leg. It was a full body hug. I laughed, not knowing what else to do.

Suddenly, the loud music stopped. The children ran to the edge of the playground and formed a single-file line. The workers were yelling at them. In unison, the children joined hands and started walking toward the brick building led by one of the workers. As the children passed, they looked back at my mom and me until they could no longer keep their balance. Some waved good-bye, others yelled, "Yo!" The girl who had grabbed my hand earlier was the last one in line. She didn't want to go inside yet and was dragging her feet. Her morose expression was familiar: It reminded me of my nursery school picture, for which I had refused to smile. The photographer had tried everything, but my expression hadn't changed. I lifted my hand to wave good-bye and smiled. The hint of a smile appeared on her face before she was yanked up the stairs.

I heard a knock on the door and jumped out of bed.

"Karen," a voice yelled. It was June. "Do you want to do it now? You're not sleeping are you?"

"No . . . no, let's do it now," I said groggily. "It'll take me a few minutes to set everything up."

"Do you want to do it in the living room?"

"Yes."

"I'll see you in there in about ten minutes then."

I struggled to clear my head. While I stumbled around the bedroom, scrambling to get all the equipment together, I thought about the questions I had prepared. Were they too much? Would June want to talk about all this? But it was too late. I would soon find out.

In the living room, I spread the legs of the Bogen tripod and adjusted them to the right height, popped the video camera on top of the tripod and attached the power supply to the back. I inserted a new two-hour tape and hooked up the lavaliere microphone. June walked in, sat on the couch and watched me as I set up her microphone. Then we began.

"Uhh," I said self-consciously, "could you talk about how and when I came here to the orphanage and the situation surrounding it?"

"Oh, let's see. I think it was 1969 . . . or was it 1970? I'm not sure. I know that you were left at the provincial city hall here in Chechon and . . . uh . . . gosh, if I had known that you were going to ask these specific questions, I would have brought your card with me." There it was again. The card. She had mentioned it earlier, but I still didn't know what it was.

"But let me try 'cause I'm all hooked up and everything." I wanted to stop and tell her to get the card, but I didn't say anything.

"I believe it was the social worker from the city hall who brought you here."

"And . . . what happened? What did she say?"

She paused for a long time. "Oh, I wish I would have known," she told me again. "I'm going to have to get it after all," she continued, fumbling with the microphone.

When June returned to the couch, the white index card floated between her fingers, playing with my mind. This is what I had traveled all this distance for, I thought. I could have just as easily obtained this information over the phone. It had literally been a phone call away all these years. This was all it would come down to: not a file, bursting with piles of confidential documents, secured in a fire-proof safety cabinet locked away in a cavernous vault—but an index card.

June had simply walked into her office, opened a small card file, looked my name up and pulled my card out. I began to feel angry. Why did so much of the adoption process seem to be about hiding information? Why hadn't this card traveled with me? Wasn't it my right to carry what little history I had with me to my new life? Why did it have to turn into a difficult and complex journey to find one damn card? Finally, I quit asking myself questions and just listened.

"Okay. Let's see what we have here." June adjusted her glasses so that they teetered on the end of her nose. After taking a deep breath, she said, "All right, someone found you at the city hall and they brought you . . . and that's all I have here is 'they,' you know, and it doesn't say who 'they' are. I assume it was a social worker there who brought you over here. It was February 19, 1969. You were almost a year old. And you were really dirty when they dropped you off. We had to give you a bath right away.

"Um . . . they said that your mother had died and no one knew where your father was. I remember that you just clung to me when you got here. You know how you can just tell sometimes when babies are insecure. You were really scared, and you wouldn't let go of me. That's why we tried to get you adopted right away. I know when a child will get attached to me really fast. I can just feel it. And I knew that if you stayed in the orphanage for too long it would be really traumatic for you to leave. So, you were only here for eight months."

I wondered whether I wanted to hear this. One thing was true: Whenever I had thought about searching for my birth parents I thought only of my birth mother. I never imagined a reunion with my father. So when June said "your mother had died," the energy I had accumulated for a search began to dissipate. I didn't know why I wasn't interested in searching for my father. Maybe it was because I connected fatherhood to my white adoptive father, from whom I was growing more and more distant.

For now, I could only try to deal with the fact that my mother was probably dead. The urge to cry was overwhelming. But a voice inside my head kept saying, "Karen, don't cry, don't cry. It won't help, you know." And I knew whose voice it was. It was my mother's. I tried so hard to remain strong, to show everyone and to prove to myself that I could handle this, that I was ready and that my expectations hadn't been shattered. I locked it all inside, trapping it indefinitely. I tightened my entire body to control the heaves that threatened to overtake me.

Tonight, I look at my hands and I wonder where they came from. They don't seem like a part of my body. They are merely a foreign attachment. I try to imagine them being in Korea, at the orphanage. But when I think of Korea, I think of another person, returning to her birthplace. Even though I am here now, writing about it, it couldn't have been me. I still don't really think of myself as an adopted person.

I look at the photograph wedged into the border of my vanity mirror. My brother, my mother, and me. My mother's aging face reminds me of her nervous expressions and mannerisms while at the orphanage. What she must have gone through to accompany me. It must have been difficult for her. But we have never talked about it. Neither there nor here. She only speaks about the trip as a "really good time, really fun, and won't we do it again?" Neither of us ever cried at the orphanage. Before we left for Korea, I had feared crying. It symbolized chaos to me, a tangible loss of control. I didn't want to be out of control, at the orphanage, with my mother. I managed to hold back all the tears. I never let go. I was always guarded, straining to block my emotions, biting my lips forcefully. Ironically, I think my mother wanted me to cry this time. I think she wanted us to cry together so that she could hug me and console me just like any mother would.

We all live behind our masks, unable to express who we really are. I wanted to prove to her that I didn't expect anything, that I wasn't disappointed at what we did or didn't find. I wanted to show her how strong I was, to make her proud I could hold back my tears, that I wasn't just thinking of myself. But this *was* my time to be selfish. And I realize I can no longer hold back these tears. I must relive that time in a way that brings some kind of harmony to my life. I must release myself in order to achieve some kind of meaningful closure. Now when I am alone, I let the tears take over, relieved that I can finally mourn.

KAI JACKSON AND
CATHERINE E. MCKINLEY
Sisters: A Reunion Story

Kai Jackson

I met Cathy when I was seventeen years old, in the Spring of 1985, the same year my mother was dying of cancer. In one of my mother's last acts of willful determination, she sent me off to the open house at the college I would be attending that fall. She gave orders from her hospital bed, insisting that I bring my tweed suit to her for inspection, arranging with an older woman relative to accompany me on the trip from Chicago to New York, soliciting aunts and uncles for the plane and hotel fare she could not afford. My mother kissed me and wished me well as I went off. Now, I imagine that one of her silent prayers was for me to meet a friend when I got there, one who would watch out for me in her absence.

I met Cathy at the open house; she was also a prospective student. I remember how awkward, excited and overwhelmed I felt that day, how filled with the new sights and smells of independent college life I was as I toured the campus with all the other students. Cathy's was an instantly familiar face because hers was like my own, so near white it could fool some people, make other people ask questions. In Cathy, I recognized the particular flair and fire I associate with blackness. I remember her close-cut naturally curly hair style, her worn jeans and brilliant red sweater. Most of all, I remember her outrageously red alligator-skin shoes. Although Cathy said little to me that day, there was a defiant drama to her that spoke of islands, East Coast chic, drumbeats and soul. At the same time I admired Cathy and wanted to be her friend, I was also wary of her. I was uncomfortable and resentful at a reminder of a painful truth in myself.

I, like Cathy, have a biracial heritage. The product of a Black mother and a white father, I was adopted when I was six months old by Black parents, Edgar

Constantine Jackson and Thomaline Francis Jackson. I have a younger brother, Cort Andrew, who is also adopted. My parents divorced when I was five. The skin colors of their children marked unspoken divisions and alliances between them. My brother is dark chocolate brown like my mother. My father was yellow-light, and although I was still lighter, I resembled him enough (we both had freckles) that people used to remark how my daddy "couldn't deny me if he tried."

My parents had always been very open with my brother and me about the fact that we were adopted. We grew up on the south side of Chicago on an all-Black boulevard street. I was raised inside the rhythms and textures of Black life. My parents were both jazz enthusiasts; their music, movements and words were a melding of their rural-South and northern-city backgrounds. They taught me I was Black, told us it was nobody else's business how we got here. My brother and I had big fun with kids who tried to figure out how we could be brother and sister, look so different from one another and be six months apart in age. "Are ya'll twins? Half-brother and sister? Step-brother and sister?" We shook our heads no and laughed to ourselves. Our private game, but also a private shame, something we kept hidden from our friends.

My mother raised us, and from her I learned the legacy of strength and endurance of Black women: "Don't depend on anybody but yourself," she said. She told me to keep my head high and to ignore kids who teased me and called me "Casper," "whitey," and "honkey." I felt our difference when I was growing up, especially in our beauty rituals: hair oil and a perm for her, setting spray and relentless combing of tangles for me. My hair was just one of the ways I felt like an outsider in my family and community; there were so many I had no words to name them.

I was twelve when I found out I was biracial. "I thought you knew," my cousin said in response to my shock. I had naively believed that light skin color had nothing to do with being mixed. "Black is what you are inside," my mother told me over and over. Now, I stood in front of the mirror for hours, looking at my face and my body and trying to figure out what part of me was "mixed." I was mad at my parents for not telling me the whole truth. Later on, I found my family history sheet from the adoption agency in my mother's file cabinet. All of the identifying information was marked out with black marker, but under "Mother," was "Black, sixteen years old," and under "Father," "Caucasian, sixteen years old." I never mentioned my discovery to my parents, and from that point on, like being adopted, I kept my knowledge of my biracial identity a secret.

When I met Cathy that spring, I looked into myself, a self I feared, was ashamed of and yet wanted to love. Because we both requested Black roommates, the college placed us together. That summer Cathy and I wrote letters of introduction to each other. I was grieving from my mother's recent death, and for the first time, I wrote of my adoptee, biracial identity. Our letters were fragile, love it or leave it testimonies of who we were: daughters of biracial unions; adopted daughters; young women and creative artists searching for definitive connection to the Black community. I was so surprised to learn of our similar backgrounds; never before had I met anyone who shared my biracial, adoptee heritage. On top of that, here was a young sister as passionately interested in writing and Black women's literature as I was. Our commonalities excited me, and I put aside my initial wariness.

Cathy and I were inseparable in our early college days. We were part of a three-percent minority of Blacks on campus, aliens in an alien world. We met a few other Black women students on campus who were also biracial and adopted. I felt my historical significance for the first time, that we might be a product of the 1960s, part of a failed experiment in hippie "free love." In college, I began to learn how American social policy had robbed me of knowledge of two crucial heritages . . . my contemporary biological and my ancient African. I came to view myself, and all Black adoptees, as "double victims" of a country that has historically disregarded the right of such people to know the full truth of our personal histories. Cathy and I struggled with these painful truths on campus; those were the days spent discovering and affirming ourselves as Black women. Together, we were a fortress against people who dared to question the authenticity of our Blackness. We decorated our room with Black art, read, talked and argued about Black books, films and political philosophy. We struggled with our boyfriends and confessed our attraction to dark-skinned, street-macho men as a means of connecting to the community. We helped start the Black student group at our college, working to bring more Black faculty and Black studies courses to the campus. My most precious coming-of-age memories are inextricably intertwined with my sister-friend Cathy.

Several years have passed since Cathy and I graduated from college, and we now live in different cities. Even though we talk on the phone at least once a week, I miss Cathy terribly. There is nothing like a good sister-friend, one who shares a similar history and life vision. I know Cathy still crunches down on the pavements of the city, seeking truth, shunning mediocrity, demanding excellence, always with a critical, focused eye. I look forward to our phone calls, where we still discuss books, politics and personal issues with honesty and passion. Most recently, I was reminded of our profound friendship on my wedding day. Our love and friendship were affirmed as I felt Cathy's support for me, and her happiness over my embracing a new level of family and belonging. I look forward to our continuously sharing our writing and other creative works, to enjoying yearly visits, to going through career-changes, midlife crises, menopause and retirement, and even to being ghosts together.

Just after my father died, I remarked to one of my favorite professors that I really had no family. I will never forget her words: "You are lucky then. You can invent some." Indeed, I believe Cathy and I have invented family in each other. We both understand, without necessarily speaking aloud, these questions that plague us and many other children of adoption: Who am I, and where did I come from? Where do I fit in? Why did you leave me? Because adoption is often mired in shame and silence, sharing stories and bonding among adoptees is life-crucial and empowering. I know that Cathy understands and identifies with the heaviness of these unanswered questions, the painful reality of personal rejection, of being helpless as our birth mothers gave us away. Cathy and I are attempting to tackle this pain by searching for our biological parents. First on my list is finding my birth mother. In Cathy, I have a friend who understands the unique importance of the mother to the Black adopted woman-child. My birth mother is my closest link, another piece in the puzzle of my woman-self.

I also look forward to meeting my birth father. For a long time, I denied the reality of my birth father: He was a source of shame in my life, proof positive of the whiteness that had kept me in tension with my Black community. I realize now he is a part of me I must embrace in order to love all of me.

For many biracial adoptees, the process of positive self-identity is complicated by color prejudices inside Black and white communities. For me, I have chosen an identity that speaks to my biological, adoptive and cultural reality; I am a Black biracial woman because I grew up amidst Black family and community—this is the framework I love and know. I have been lucky to have Cathy in my life, my mirror sister spirit, a friend whose adoption experiences give me perspective and support for my own life journey.

Catherine E. McKinley

Kai stood before me as my mirror image: so light-skinned that one immediately played the racial guessing game, much like the one *Ebony* magazine ran periodically in the 1970s and early 1980s: "Who's Black?" was the caption above the rows of variously hued and configured faces. I recognized so much of myself in her soft, close-cut hair—not "nappy" in the classic sense, but resistant of both fine-tooth and straightening combs; her formal wool suit and small wire glasses; and the somewhat tentative, self-conscious assertion of a Black woman-self in her manners, attitude and speech. When I met Kai in the spring of 1985, at Admitted Students' Day, at the college we would attend, I felt a sense of *anger* that was so markedly different from the eager excitement I felt connecting with the other six or so entering Black students. I hated her. Most pointedly, in her, I confronted myself and my raging pain and anxieties. I had never looked into the eyes of someone who so closely mirrored me, not knowing any blood kin, and living the formative years of my life with the painful absence of self-images.

I was raised in a small factory town in Massachusetts that was predominantly white, working class, and devoutly Roman Catholic. There were less than a handful of Black persons living there. Upon rare sighting of another one of "us," I would stand in my tracks, watching intently for some proof of my belonging. However, they were not "Black" like me, which many considered not "Black" at all. Nor did they live on the Hill, as I did, but on the other side of downtown, literally over the tracks and past the industrial parks. They were mostly elderly women and men, remnants of an earlier era. Hosted by relatives, their children and grandchildren had attended schools in the South or the not-so-distant Boston neighborhoods of Roxbury and Mattapan and never seemed to return "home." The only really sizeable groups of non-white people in town were recently arrived Vietnamese and Laotian refugees and I was separated from them by class, language, culture and political circumstance.

My adoptive family is quite plainly white Anglo-Saxon Protestants and New Englanders. Despite their assumed belonging, our family stood in stark relief against others in the community. I thought of us as being like the Addams family: creating public stirs, my parents seemingly unconscious and certainly not greatly caring of how their values set us apart. We lived in a dilapidated house, encased in foliage in the midst of neighbors with obsessively manicured homes, one or two generations removed from factory piece-work, and caught up in all of the material displays of class consciousness. I saw myself as Thing, a freak, feeling much like an appendage to my family—solitary, truncated, grasping. They moved there, they would admit, naively expecting the town would become integrated as Black Bostonians "realized Martin Luther King Jr.'s dream" and became commuters.

My mother is a hearty woman—independent, forthright in manner and decidedly unconcerned with the conventional trappings of "womanhood." "There goes your Dad!" someone would yell as my mother bicycled or roller-skated by, her engineers cap pulled down over her ears. My father—a towering, gentle, even-tempered and emotionally reserved man—has been my mother's true partner of thirty-five years.

My brother, two years older than me, is also adopted, however his straw-blond hair and blue eyes are not obvious markers of difference. They run in the family. And now, as if he were my father's biological son, he is "darkening" and balding well before thirty. As a child he was sensitive, what others have thought of as eccentric—and physically reckless—always stitched up as a result of some fantastic feat. At an early age, with our growing consciousness of race and gender divisions, we separated along the distinct lines of difference drawn between us.

I am of mixed-parentage, but I never saw myself as biracial. The one-drop rule reigned for my generation. Mixed was not an identity. I would never have chosen this nor would others have allowed it. You stood in the face of insistence by both Blacks and whites that you were the "other" nigger.

I've come to understand that conceptions of Blackness and identity are relative to one's context, constantly shifting and threatening to batter you in the throws. In the town in which I was raised, I was the Black child: "porch monkey," "jungle bunny." My skin was "dark" and my hair was braided "afro-turf." In Black communities outside, I discovered I was "yellow" with "white girl's hair." To others, I become a generic brown. In my current Brooklyn neighborhood, Latinos, South Asians, Arabs, and even Jews routinely nod to me in recognition. And so I realize that the questions and privileges, the stigmas and struggles that defined my youth would have been very different if the context were even slightly altered. Knowing this dulls the sharp edges of my childhood.

Kai and I were placed as roommates that fall. We were the only two entering students who explicitly requested to share a room with another Black student. We wrote to each other several times during the summer before we left for college. The woman I met on the page began to slowly break through my anger. I could not resist her offer of friendship.

Kai's mother had just died of cancer, and her father had had a massive stroke a month or so following her death. I connected very strongly with her sense of loss, and what I imagined was liberation from the constraints of family. She wrote also of her love of books and her new passion for Black women's writing, which I couldn't ignore. Discovering Black literature, and particularly Black feminist writing, provided me with a provocative, yet in many ways comfortable, socialization. As a sister outsider, I had books and my own writing to affirm my belonging and allowing me to stretch into myself.

Kai's early forthrightness about being biracial and adopted startled me, as I had hidden this about myself as best I could. I denied being biracial to anyone who asked, relying on rhetoric, insisting that all African Americans are racially mixed. I would walk as far ahead of my mother as possible without seeming to disrespect her or causing her to call out to me, foiling my attempts to disown her. Once I left home, as I did to attend boarding school, I risked "coming out" as an adoptee only when that terrifying moment of truth ("Your parent's are here!") collided with the elaborate and painfully transparent fantasies I'd constructed about who I was.

Despite the intense connection I felt to Kai, I still wrestled with my anger at her image and with my jealousy at her having a "legitimate" tie through her family to her Blackness.

What I remember most poignantly from Kai's and my college days are the frequent journeys we made on the Metro-North trains to Manhattan. Twenty minutes to 125th Street! We rode those trains at dawn, returning from a night of clubbing, or in the late afternoon after freshman seminar, on schedule with the domestic workers and other laborers traveling between Westchester and the Bronx and Harlem. I would survey each Black face, for some resemblance to my own. Kai also did this, searching both for her birth mother and the one deceased, hoping she lived among us in some altered form. We were always boarding the train in search of community and an "authentic" experience of ourselves, transformed into sisters/sistahs. It was so wonderful to hear "Hello, my sisters!" boom out at us on the uptown streets. No one challenged our belonging. We were frequently asked if we were twins, which we never denied, although we look *so* different and I stand at least five inches above her. Passing felt so sublime. For a short time we could live our yearnings.

Kai and I came to political consciousness together, embracing and struggling with both pretty radical and narrow ideologies. We weighed our burgeoning ideas and identities against everything we encountered. We were campus critics and self-styled "militants." And we traversed some incredible emotional borders together, breaking many silences around adoption and our experiences. Our intense need for recognition as conscious Black women and as adoptees is what cements our sisterhood.

My relationship with Kai helped me to understand, and today reminds me at moments when feelings of alienation creep over me, that our experiences are precisely what holds us to "the Black community," rather than pushing us outside of it, whether or not others recognize this.

Our experiences, though in some ways unique, are intimately tied to the lives of other Black women in our struggle for selfhood and freedom from the narrowly drawn lines of race. Our ten years of sisterhood have carried me to a profound level. I've learned to love Kai deeply, as I continue to reconcile my contradictory feelings about myself. I have come to love both Kai's spiritual and physical beauty, her creativity born of outsidership, and her need to claim self in a tradition of imperfect Black women—women who defy what femaleness and Blackness have been constructed as. In the absence of and perhaps in spite of any blood-kin, Kai is my sister. In some ways she feels more real to me than any other claim of family.

I've come to realize that it is this struggle with anger and love that profoundly marks my relationships to my families, both adopted, invented and unknown. This struggle has also been the basis of my emotional growth, my creative life, and what I increasingly feel is the need to vigilantly struggle against racism and the ways in which it violates and confines all persons' lives.

FLORENCE FISHER

Somebody's Child

We had not arrived home until nearly four in the morning, and I could hardly sleep. Although physically and emotionally exhausted, my mind spun with expectations. The first thing I did when I got to the office the next morning was to check the Westchester telephone directories for 1967, 1968, 1969 and 1970. There was a William B. Okun listed; and at the same address a Marsha Okun. There was a Robert L. Okun at another address. They were in all three books but not in the current directory. I still had my mother's office phone number; though they'd moved, she might still be working there. If it was a small firm or if she had a private phone, perhaps it would be she who'd answer.

"I'm sorry," a woman told me, "Mrs. Okun doesn't work here anymore."

I said: "Can you tell me where she *does* work?"

"No," the woman said hesitantly. "Who is this speaking?"

"I'm just in from California for a couple of days," I said, "and I'm not sure I have the right people, but I'm trying to trace my grandmother's family. I believe Mrs. Okun is a cousin of mine, and I'm terribly distressed because I just found out she moved from Dobbs Ferry a year ago. Can you possibly tell me where she moved?"

Editor's note: The author was born to Florence Cohen and Fred Fisher and the name *Anna Fisher* was placed on her birth certificate. When she was adopted a few months later, her adoptive parents gave her the name Florence. After completing the search and finding her parents-of-birth, the author began using her original surname. Although this is a true story, all of the names of the individuals mentioned here have been changed, with the exception of Florence Fisher and her father, Fred Fisher. This piece is excerpted from the book-length memoir: *The Search for Anna Fisher*, Arthur Fields Books, 1973.

"Oh, is that all?" the woman said. "Mrs. Okun moved to Manhattan last year."

I asked: "Does she have a daughter named Marsha?"

"Why, yes."

I now knew, for the first time, that I had a sister.

"And a son named Robert?"

"Yes, she does."

"Does she have any other children?" I asked.

"No. No more children that I know of."

When I hung up, I got out the current Manhattan directory. Okun was a great name. Smith, Jones or Cohen would have finished me! My mother and her family were all listed. She had done exactly what I'd do. She had raised her children in the suburbs and then retired to Manhattan—perhaps to be near the theater and opera. She had retired to *live*, not to die. I knew her. I also, inexplicably, had an overwhelming sense of protectiveness toward her. To me, she was still, somehow, seventeen years old; I still felt like *her* mother, and I thought, *I must protect her; I must be very careful, very tender.*

I dialed her home number. The phone rang once, twice, ten times. There was no answer. Perhaps she had another job.

I dialed Robert's number. Maybe he or his wife, if he had one, could give me another number to call. I got a busy signal and hung up impatiently. As I was going to dial again, the phone rang.

"Florence?" an excited voice said. "I've found your mother. She's in Manhattan." It was Mr. Brooks.

I said: "I've also found her."

Speaking quickly, he said: "I just called your brother's wife. You know you have a brother?" He had gotten to the office early, seen my note, and had gone through the current directories. He had found all the Okuns in Manhattan and spoken to my sister-in-law. That was why I'd gotten a busy signal.

Oh, my God, I thought. What has he done? I didn't want to hurt his feelings; he was trying to help me, and he had been one of the very few people who ever *had* helped me. He was obviously deeply interested and genuinely excited about all the sudden developments. But if my mother's family did not know of my existence I wanted to shield her.

"Mr. Brooks," I said, a quiet fear creeping into my voice. "What did you say to her?"

"Well," he said, "I told her it was imperative that I locate her mother-in-law immediately on a matter of the utmost legal importance."

I closed my eyes. It was crucial that I make the initial contact. "What did you do?" I asked.

"She took my number and said she'd give it to your mother and have her call."

"What were you planning to do then?" I asked softly.

He said: "I was going to ask your mother whether she wants to see you."

"You were going to do what?"

I told him quietly, patiently, that I appreciated with all my heart that he wanted to help me, but that I had to do this myself. I told him that my mother never had to see me again, but that I had questions and she was the only person that could answer them. I had no intention of intruding into her life, but I simply could not give her the option of *not* seeing me—not after all I'd been through.

"I only wanted to save you the aggravation," he said.

"I know, but no one can save me any aggravation. I've had it all. What else can happen? It's all over. Twenty years ago, had I been lucky enough to meet you, you could have saved me a tremendous amount of heartache. But I've gone the whole route relatively alone, and I have to finish it alone. I won't unload it on anybody else. I can handle it. If my mother tells me to go to hell I can handle it, and if she welcomes me with open arms I can handle it. If I could handle the last twenty years, I can manage whatever is coming in the next fifteen minutes."

He wished me good luck and asked me to call him later.

I jiggled the buttons on the telephone and got a fresh outside line. When my brother's wife picked up the phone, I said: "My name is Audrey. I'm from California, and I think I'm a cousin of your husband's. I understand my lawyer, Mr. Brooks, just called you."

"Oh, yes," she said. "I'm terribly disturbed about that. I was wondering whether to call my mother-in-law immediately, or speak to Robert first."

"Don't call anyone," I said. "Please don't be upset. It's all quite simple." I told her an involved story I'd fabricated, concerning "my" grandmother and Hannah Cohen. I told her I was looking for Hannah Sweik Cohen's daughter, using the English spelling of "Zweick."

"Oh, that's my husband's grandmother," she said, obviously relieved. "I remember the name Sweik. I'm so pleased it isn't something more serious."

"What I'd really like to do," I said, "is see your mother-in-law and any other relatives that I can—and be able to report back to my grandmother that I was able to make contact with her family. I have to be back in California in a few days."

"I'm so relieved," she said.

"I tried her at home and . . ."

"Oh, she's at work now."

I said: "Would you give me the number, please?"

Every moment mattered to me now. In a few hours I'd be able to reach her at home, but I wanted it all over with. Fast. I felt like someone who has been traveling down a tortuous ski slope for a long time; I wanted to get to the bottom. Also, for a number of reasons it would be better to speak to her at her office than her home.

"Of course I can give you her number," my sister-in-law said. She told me my mother worked at a large department store, in the executive office.

It didn't occur to me to wait five minutes or until I could compose myself. What was the point? I wouldn't be more composed in one hour, ten hours or ten years. I dialed each digit slowly, watching my fingers as they turned the dial clockwise to the top, all the way—each time slowly, crisply. *You're calling your mother. In another minute you'll hear your mother's voice.*

I coughed nervously to clear my throat and waited for someone to pick up at the other end. I could feel my face flushing, and I fought to keep the tears out of my voice. When the store operator answered, I said: "May I speak to Mrs. Okun, please, in the executive office?" My voice sounded calm; it had not broken.

"One moment." I heard the interoffice buzzer, lighter than the regular ring.

Then I heard, "Executive office. Mrs. Okun."

I was conscious of the way she enunciated each word. Her voice sounded— or did I imagine it?—similar to mine. I had often recorded my voice, to hear how I sang Italian love songs or the blues, and I could tell immediately that hers was a halftone down from my mezzo. But she enunciated her words in the same way.

I said: "You don't know me, Mrs. Okun, but I believe we're cousins." I heard my voice, out of the ghastly turmoil and near hysteria inside me, emerge cool and calm. I could feel myself beginning to shake all over. Was this me? Or was someone else saying the words? "My name is Audrey Orenstein," I said, "and I'm quite sure we're related."

The woman said: "We don't have any Orensteins in the family."

"That's my married name," I said. My strength grew while I talked, but I knew I'd have to maintain absolute control if I was to carry this off without her suspecting for one moment what was going on inside me. "I'm from California, and my grandmother came into the country between 1900 and 1910. She came with her cousin Hannah."

I heard my mother catch her breath. "That was my mother's name," she said tentatively.

I told her that my grandmother and her cousin were separated soon after they got to America, and that my grandmother had gone out west, where she married and had a family of her own. "She's very old and infirm now," I said, "but she still thinks nostalgically of Russia and of coming over on the boat with her cousin." I had not realized that I could maintain such outward composure. I knew all the details of my family so well that I had no trouble spinning out my tale. I didn't want to, but I knew it was necessary, and I kept hearing the words—calm and cool and pleasant—as if they were not mine. "They never saw each other again," I said. I paused for a moment. "Her cousin's name was Hannah Sweik."

"That was my mother!"

I felt horrible. My first contact with my mother was a lie. I wanted to say it now: "Mother. Mother."

But I couldn't.

It would have been monstrous to announce, after all these years, "I'm your daughter." How could I possibly tell her that over the phone?

My well rehearsed story was so plausible that she simply accepted it. *I'm lying to my mother.* I wanted to cry out. I wanted to tell her: "I'm your daughter, Mother." But I heard myself still chatting on pleasantly into the phone about Cohens and more Cohens, while inside there was this shout: *Forgive me. I don't want to deceive you. I have to do it this way.*

She was saying: "Oh, I can't tell you how excited I am. I must call a cousin of mine—and yours, too, I guess—who keeps a family tree. I *must* see you. How long will you be here?"

"Just a few days. I'm here with my husband. We've got to go back to California soon." *I don't want to lie to you, Mother.*

She said: "Let's set a time right now."

I said: "Would you meet me for lunch? Tomorrow . . ."

"I wouldn't think of meeting you for lunch," she said, interrupting me. "You and your husband must have dinner with us."

"No," I said softly. "It would be too much trouble for you." It was what I would have done. A hundred times I'd invited friends of ours from out of town to our apartment for dinner—just like that. They'd call from the airport, suddenly, and I'd go out to get them. They'd call from the city and I'd insist, and wouldn't take no's, that they come right over for dinner. But I couldn't go to her house. I couldn't possibly do that. But how could I get out of it?

"Look," she said. "I can't talk now because I'm at work and there are people in the office. Is there some place I can call you later? Are you staying at a hotel?"

I parried quickly. "No, I'm staying with relations of my husband," I said, and gave her my home phone number.

"Good," she said. "I'll call you as soon as I get home tonight, and we'll arrange a time for you to come to dinner. I can't wait to meet you, Audrey."

When she hung up, I ran to the Xerox room and broke down completely. Did I *really* have a mother? Had I *really* just spoken to her? I felt disembodied—as if I was on the outside looking in at my life. Tears poured down my cheeks, and I pressed myself against the machine and sobbed uncontrollably.

I had always been angry when a friend or acquaintance assumed that at the end of my search I'd probably find someone reprehensible. The unwed mother who gives a child up for adoption, everyone assumes, is a slut. When I was a teenager, my adoptive parents had watched every move I made; they questioned me on my social life in detail; they censored my mail; they insulted my friends. I had long since realized they had been convinced that unless they hovered over me like constant *bodyguards*, I'd wind up as my mother had. Like mother, like daughter. Heredity, for the adopted child, only works here; otherwise, in all other ways, the assumption is that the child owes everything to his environment, to his adoptive parents.

I had told my friends, "So what? I only want to find my parents; that's the important thing. I don't care if I find them in the gutter. They're what's behind the wall. They're part of the truth of who I am—and that's what I'm looking for. I'm looking for Anna Fisher."

Beyond that, though, I had always had a firm belief that I would not find my mother in the gutter. There were qualities in me that I knew I would find in her and in my father—stubbornness, tenacity, pride, a love for music and theater and life. I had spoken to a perfectly lovely woman that morning who was my mother. She had sounded so warm and generous. She was outgoing and effervescent. She was so friendly, so kind.

All that afternoon I kept asking myself: "Did I really talk to my mother?" Yes, it *had* been her. I had done it.

And I had beaten the sealed records. I had beaten the system; they had sealed my records, but they couldn't seal my mind. The satisfaction I had in this was all I really had—until I actually saw my mother. There was nothing more anyone could do to me, ever. All afternoon, intermittently, I cried and laughed and thought of what I would have to do next.

I cried on the subway, and the rush-hour crowd must have thought me stark mad. An elderly lady put her hand on my shoulder and said: "Can I help you, dear?"

"No," I said, smiling broadly. "I found my mother."

I cried in the butcher shop, and the butcher, an old friend said: "What's the matter? Are you all right?"

"I spoke to my mother," I told him.

He knew about my search. "She found her mother," he said excitedly to a customer, and the woman, seeing my joy, not knowing anything about the circumstances, put her arms around me and held me tight.

The phone was ringing when I entered my apartment a half hour later. I left the key in the door, dropped my packages and ran into the bedroom.

"Hello, is this Audrey?" I knew the voice immediately.

"Yes," I said calmly.

"This is Florence Okun." *My God, if you only knew who you were talking to.* "You know, I've just called my cousin," she said, "and it's so strange: She keeps such a fantastic account of the family's activities but she's never heard of you or your family."

I said: "I never knew there was family in New York either." How could I keep so calm? I was holding the phone with my left hand and holding my left hand with my right hand to keep the receiver from knocking against my teeth.

We laughed and chatted and both sounded so self-assured, and it was all very light-headed and happy and otherworldly. I heard myself say: "I'd love to know something about your family."

"Oh, I have a wonderful family," she told me. She spoke glowingly about her son and daughter, about their achievements. Her son had majored in music and now was a performer.

I was starved for details and listened avidly as she went on to tell me about her daughter's academic honors, her son's plans for the future, and how pleased she was with her daughter-in-law. "So you see," she said at length, "I have two lovely children."

I could tell she liked talking to me. I heard her say: "Our house was always filled with children and music."

It was almost too much to bear. I was sitting on the bed, the receiver pressed so close to my ear that my ear had grown flushed and hot. Outside the window, I could see a bright June sunset forming above the New Jersey Palisades. Already the pinks and blues, the gold and red were reflected on the Hudson River.

It was all so unreal. I wanted to say: *I'm your daughter. You have three children.*

She was telling me about her brother, respected in his profession. My uncle. I felt sick deceiving her. She was being so open with me, so unsuspecting. *But I have a right to this information*, I thought. *It's my life history, too. This is* my *family. I have a right to know what my brother is, what my*

*sister is. I have a right to know and feel proud of what an uncle of mine, my
mother's brother, has achieved.*

Without resentment, but wistfully, I let my feelings speak. *We would have
been close as mother and daughter I know it. . . .* But I cut these thoughts off
in a moment. What was, was. You couldn't go back.

"How proud you must be," I said.

"I am."

I once had Sodium Pentothal for an operation. When I came out of it,
I heard everything through a mist. I felt that way now. Was I dreaming it
all? It was too impossible: me talking to my mother, listening to her tell me
about my brother and sister; she, chatting on as if we were old friends. The
deception, the joy, the wistful sadness. And all the while I kept watching the
bright orange crest of the sun slip down slowly into the Palisades: now crim-
son purple, now pink and robin's-egg blue, as it vanished further below the
slowly drifting clouds. Would she vanish too? Was she real?

"I have to work until five-thirty," she said, "but I want you and your husband to come to dinner tomorrow night."

I asked: "Why did you move to New York last year? Didn't you like the
suburbs?"

"Not really," she said. "But we made the decision for the children, while
they were growing up, and now I want to be near the theater and the concert
halls. I love Manhattan. Will tomorrow night be all right for you both?"

"Oh, by the way," I said, changing the subject again. "I've moved around
the country quite a bit. Have you always lived in this area? Your accent isn't
New York."

She laughed and said: "I've always tried to speak properly."

"Have you lived in New York all your life?" I pressed.

She paused. I could feel a painful silence. "Yes," she said hesitantly. She
paused again. "Except for the time between when I was fourteen and seventeen. We lived in . . . in Philadelphia for a while. Look, I love having people
for dinner, and I wouldn't think of letting you leave town without coming
over. We can try to figure out why the family tree isn't what it should be. I
want you and your husband to come . . . let's make tomorrow definite."

"Well, we only have a few days . . . so why don't I simply meet you for
lunch?"

"No, I'd really like to make it for dinner, when we'll have time to sit down
for several hours and not be rushed. Anyway, my daughter is getting married
and I'm going for fittings on my dress during lunch hours."

If her husband and family didn't know, it could blow her life apart to tell
her in front of them, or anywhere near them. I *had* to see her alone. *Even if*

I go, I thought rapidly, *maybe she looks like me; maybe she's a dead ringer for me and everyone will see it. There aren't so many years separating us.* The hypocrisy, the deception, were beyond my strength.

"Please say you'll come," she said.

"Can we have a drink together after you finish work?"

"That's silly. I only live a block from my office."

I said: "Perhaps a quick cup of coffee?" I was beginning to sound foolish. She couldn't help noticing if I kept this up.

"Absolutely not. I won't hear of anything else. You *must* come for dinner."

"Thank you," I said, "of course we'll come. You're very persuasive." I knew I couldn't push her further. Tomorrow I'd handle it. But no way, anyway, would I go to her house. "Why don't I meet you at your office and go home with you?"

She seemed puzzled by this, but we finally agreed, and I promised to meet her the next day at five-thirty.

We had been talking for more than an hour. After I hung up I sat on the bed watching the last Monet-like moments of the sunset. The cars going back and forth on the George Washington Bridge turned on their lights, and the crisscross movement, back and forth across the river, was like the electrical current between two poles.

The fantasy of the evening turned into a long night, crowded with tossing and nightmares, until all disappeared in exhausted sleep.

I had so much wanted to look pretty, but the rain seemed only to increase as I ran out to hail a cab; I was afraid that despite my raincoat and plastic rain bonnet, I'd look a mess by the time I saw her. In the cab I realized that though my arms were calm, my legs were still shaking. I kept thinking: *How do I say, I'm your daughter. How do I say the words? And where?*

I told the cab driver: "Please hurry. But please be careful." Don't let anything happen to me before I see my mother. I looked at my face in a hand mirror. My eyes were still red and a little swollen. I put on dark glasses.

It was good that I'd left early. We were in the midst of rush-hour traffic and for long minutes we'd stay in one place, listening to the incessant honking, watching the windshield wipers snap back and forth, back and forth. *How do I say it?*

I had to talk to someone or I'd burst. "I'm going to see my mother," I said out loud, "for the first time in my life."

The cab driver, a burly man with a peaked cap flat on his head, turned around, looked at me, and said: "Whaddaya mean yer gonna see your mother for the first time?"

I leaned forward. "I was adopted. I've looked for her all my life, and only found her yesterday. She doesn't know I'm coming; she doesn't know I'm her daughter."

When we stopped in another traffic jam a few moments later, he turned around again, looked at me, and could only shake his head. *What will she look like? What will she say? Will she be able to take the shock?* I noticed that my hands were gripping the door handle with a death-hold; they were like ice.

The cab driver said: "That's some story, lady. I've heard lotsa stories, but that's *some* story."

In a few more minutes we were there. As I handed the driver his money, he turned around again, saying in a husky voice: "Good luck, honey."

"Thanks," I said. "I'll need it."

With the rain bonnet and dark glasses obscuring my face, I walked into the store, found an information booth and asked where the executive offices were. Upstairs I asked the way to Mrs. Okun's office.

"Through that door," a clerk said. "Do you have an appointment?"

I said: "She's expecting me."

I pushed the door and, following it as it swung inward, thought, *This is it.*

The first thing I saw were my mother's legs: They were plump. She was bending over some files, and as I saw her I thought, *That's what I'm going to look like in seventeen years.* She was small—like me—but heavier, as I'd be if I didn't eat lettuce.

She turned around.

I have never known nor will I ever feel again a wave of happiness such as I did the moment I first saw my mother. She was no longer a dream, an idea, a figment of my imagination; she was not an image conjured up by my longing, a shadow haunting my sleep. My mother was real.

In an instant I took in every feature of her face: her eyes, her high cheekbones, a certain curve of her ears, the precise shape of her nose, her expression. Only her mouth was different, and she was heavier; otherwise we might have been sisters. Even her hair was dark, my natural color; the shape of the face and the animation in her eyes were the same as mine. She was not pretty, not glamorous—nor am I.

Suddenly the anguish of years fell away.

I had grown so used to the heaviness in my heart, had lived with the pain for so long, that when it fell away I felt light and free.

She said to me: "Are you Audrey?"

I said: "Yes, I am."

"Would you mind waiting a moment, dear?" she asked.

A moment? I had an impulse to laugh hysterically. From behind my dark glasses, from under my hoodlike rain bonnet, I peered out at her. I memorized every line of her face. *A moment!* I'd waited years, waited in courts and lawyers' offices, waited while strangers scratched their memories, waited for names to appear in dry old telephone directories. *Yes, I could wait a moment longer. Now, mother, I can wait.* "No," I said. "Of course I don't mind waiting."

Maybe it was the drug I'd taken. I felt light. I sat in the outer office, waiting for my mother to come out, and thought of the countless hours I had spent at my other mother's kidney-shaped dressing table with the three mirrors, looking at all those family pictures, trying desperately to find a nose or eye or ear among the hundreds of old photographs that reminded *me* of *me*. *How do I tell her?* There was so very much I wanted to say to her; I wanted to tell her how happy I was, just seeing her, just talking to her—but I couldn't think of the right first words.

I loved the way she looked. She *was* my mother. The real shock was seeing that she wasn't seventeen years old, as I had been imagining her; but there was absolutely no doubt in my mind who she was.

In a few moments she came out, carrying her umbrella and saying, "I'm ready."

I'm not, I thought. I had an intense desire to touch her.

Soon we were in the elevator making idle conversation. I could scarcely hear anything she said. I wanted to take off my dark glasses but did not. I knew I couldn't tell her here, in a crowded elevator. But where? We were nearing the first floor, and I knew we'd only have a block before we reached her house. I had to find a way to stop, and to stop her.

Outside, the storm had grown heavier. We looked at each other and shook our heads. She opened her umbrella; I opened mine.

We started walking up the block. Thoughts crowded my mind as I searched for a way out of the trap. *I've got to stop her. I can't go home.* I turned to her and started to speak but did not.

She said something about the rain, something about a casserole in the oven, something about having gone home at lunchtime to prepare something. I heard her words, but I couldn't catch hold of them. My mind was working too fast.

We had gone a block when I took a quick breath and said: "I wonder if we could go somewhere for coffee before we go to your house."

She gave me a curious look and said: "We could have it at my home."

I said, "There's something I'd like to ask you about both our families that . . . that really doesn't concern your husband or mine. So could we just have a few moments together—before we go to your house? Please?"

She looked at me strangely again, skeptically, and said: "Of course. If you want to. There's a coffee shop down the block."

We walked toward it, saying nothing now. We closed our umbrellas, went in, walked down past the counter and found a table in the back. In a moment we were seated.

She looked at me expectantly.

I wanted desperately to say something to her, anything. A full minute or two went by. I could tell that the tranquilizer had stopped working. She kept looking at me; I still had on my dark glasses and hooded rain bonnet, and peered out from under them at her.

I said: "I don't know how . . . to begin."

I choked up. I didn't want to cry. *Oh God, don't let me break down and cry*.

She said nothing. I *couldn't* tell her; the words would not come out of my mouth. I opened my purse quickly, fumbled in it, looked down and took out my birth certificate. I handed the paper across the table to her. Then I took out the Order of Adoption, her birth certificate, her marriage license and then the two death certificates of Moishe Cohen and Hannah Zweick Cohen. One by one I handed them to her.

Neither of us said a word. Her face, looking briefly at the birth certificate and then toward me, was blank. I removed my rain bonnet, folded it and laid it on the table. I removed my dark glasses and put them in my purse. I looked constantly at her face. It was a mask.

She took all the papers in her hands now and, very casually, very quickly flipped through them with her fingers, glancing briefly at each one. Then she put them down.

A stranger would have been more interested in reading them. My mother *knew* the contents.

I said: "I want you to know that I don't have any desire to intrude in your life but . . ."

She looked directly at me and, without changing her expression, said: "What is this?"

I said quietly: "I've spent the last twenty years looking for you." I looked at her. The cousin who had been so delighted to take a cousin home to dinner had vanished. Her expression had become cool, veiled. "It should be obvious that I don't want to intrude in your life or I would have gone right to your home. But I've been searching all my life, my whole life, and there are questions that I have that only two people in the world can answer—you and my father."

She looked directly at me, and without a moment's hesitation said: "I believe you're mistaken. I'm not the person you're looking for."

Did she really say that?

Was it possible?

She took out a cigarette, lit it and began to smoke rapidly. The waitress standing beside our table asked us impatiently what we wanted to order. We both said "coffee" at the same time.

Did she really say that?

I told her I had been adopted as a baby. I felt ridiculous. I told her there were many things in my nature that I could in no way attribute to my environment.

"I've always felt it was a person's environment that made them what they are," she said.

"It's because I'm so different genetically from my adoptive parents . . . this above all led me to search for my father—and for you."

"I'm terribly sorry," she said, "but I'm really not the person you're looking for." She lit another cigarette.

I looked at her but said nothing. She saw I was not going to drop it.

She asked: "Why is this so important to you? It's not the mother who bears you," she said, "but the one who brings you up who counts." *That* from my mother, too. Did she *really* believe it? Or was it a bitter, but necessary, rationalization for what she had done?

"I didn't look only for my mother and my father. I looked for the truth. I've been lied to all my life. I have a right to the truth and there are only two people in the world who can give it to me. Until I find my father, there's only you. Nobody else."

She must *find it in her heart to tell me.*

She finished her fourth or fifth cigarette and ground it into an ashtray.

"The truth," I said softly, "that's all I want from you. Nothing else. I don't want to be included in your life. That would be nice, but if it's not possible, it's not possible; I have a good life. But I must have the answers. I want to know who my father was. I want to know why I was given up for adoption. I want to know who you are. I want to know what you are. I want to know who and what my grandparents were."

I was speaking in a low, soft tone. I did not want to badger her like this. "I have a child," I said, "and I have a responsibility to pass this information on to him, just as you have to pass it on to me. I must have these answers—for my peace of mind. I've earned the answers."

She said: "I wish I could help you, but I can't."

I said: "You can if you want to."

She asked me to tell her something about myself, what I did.

I told her that I lived in New York not California; that I simply couldn't tell her on the phone who I was. "The very fact that I called my brother's wife and gave her the same story should prove to you that I don't wish to hurt you." I told her why I didn't want to come to her house. "I couldn't sit at your table," I said, "and look at your husband—not knowing if he knew—and pretend to be your cousin. When I'm your child."

She lit another cigarette and began to ask me questions—who I was, what I'd done with my life.

It was bizarre. Either she *was* my mother or she wasn't my mother. If she wasn't, why would she ask all these questions? Why would she be interested?

I had seen nothing but a studied calm in her eyes. She sat there looking at *me* with *my* face. If she was bluffing, no one had ever done it better. But was it possible, even remotely possible, that she *wasn't* my mother?

I had checked and checked—a hundred times—those documents that now lay before her on the table, those papers she had flipped through so casually. Could there be any doubt whatsoever that the woman before me, who looked like me and spoke like me, was not Florence Cohen, the daughter of Morris and Hannah Sweik Cohen, the wife of Frederick Fisher? Was it remotely possible that some false names were placed on my birth certificate, and that I had checked out a family for twenty years that was no more mine than a stranger's?

I decided to answer her questions.

I told her I'd always had a passion for reading; I told her I loved music and the arts and the theater, that I'd always been something of a dreamer. I told her I loved to make things with my hands, and that I'd been taking music lessons and voice lessons and that I sang in a semiprofessional chorus. "I love to sing," I told her, "and to play the piano. I've even taught myself several languages."

She looked at me and for a moment I thought—or I may have imagined it—that a glimmer came into her eyes. For a moment they seemed not so masked, so cool. Was it pride? Did she recognize in my face and my loves something of her own? Did she see in my interests something that might have been born in her? She kept smoking incessantly, one cigarette after the other, lighting one with the other.

She casually picked up the documents again, glanced through them and said: "I *couldn't* be the person you're looking for; I was born in 1920."

She flipped them until she came to Hannah Cohen's death certificate. "My mother's name was spelled Z-w-e-i-k," she said, pronouncing the word carefully. "Without the *c*. I really wish I could help you," she said quickly, "but I can't."

I took a deep breath now. I had wanted to spare her. I saw no reason to hurt her. All I wanted, for once, was the truth. I was getting lies again—and now from *her*. *Am I asking you for so much?* I thought. *You want to know about my life. All right. I'm going to let you know about my life. I love you; you're my mother, but . . .*

And then, blow by blow, without embellishment, I told her what my life had been as a child.

"And still," I said quietly, when I had finished, "that is not the reason I looked. I don't resent *you* because of it: I looked because there was a closed door that I had to open. Only you have the key."

I had no more strength. I had nothing else to say. She had listened to every word; she had looked at the documents; she had watched me constantly, looking down only now and then at her cigarette or at her hands—chubby little hands, like mine.

I can be just as cool when I have to. "*Il sangue chiama*," the Italians say. Blood calls blood. Maybe not. I can be cool—but could I deny my own child?

I was numb. I could go on no longer. I gave an enormous sigh and settled back in my chair. *Basta*. Enough.

She put out her last cigarette, stood up and said for the third time: "I'm sorry, I'm not the person you're looking for." *She never said, "I'm not your mother."*

I saw, as she picked up the check for the two cups of coffee we hadn't touched, that her hands were shaking now. I had wanted to get to the check first, but I couldn't move my arms.

She took out her change. I thought, *Let your mother buy you a cup of coffee, Florence.* Then she knocked over the ashtray, did not turn back and hurried out.

I sat at the table unable to move. *Well*, I thought, *there goes my mother.*

I ordered a cup of tea but didn't drink it. I looked at the little pile of documents on the table, where my mother had left them. I sat for half an hour, unable to move, unable, really, to think. Finally I tried to compose myself. Stan was waiting and he'd be worried. I reached across the table, took the papers in my hand and slowly put them back in my purse. As I got up to leave I noticed the fallen ashtray and bent down to pick it up.

On the floor, next to the ashtray, was something black.

I stared at it.

She had dropped her wallet.

It was too late to go after her, and I certainly didn't want to leave it with the people at the luncheonette. I *couldn't* bring it to her home. So I took it with me.

The first thing I said to my husband was: "She said, 'I'm not the person you're looking for.' "

I took her wallet out of my purse and placed it on the table.

"What's that?" Stan asked.

"Her wallet. She dropped it."

He asked: "Have you looked in it?"

"No," I said. I was obsessed with privacy. I didn't even glance at the other side of my husband's postcards.

But I knew I had to see what was in this wallet. *Maybe she's not your mother,* I thought. *It's not possible, but she did say she was born in a different year.* Inside the wallet would I find the final proof? Stan looked at me when I picked it up, and nodded.

The first item I saw was her driver's license. It gave her correct day of birth, and the year was the same as that on her birth certificate. There was a signature. I took the documents out from my purse, laid them on the table and fetched out one I was searching for.

Her signature, forty years later, was nearly identical to that on the wedding license.

JACKIE KAY

The Adoption Papers

In *The Adoption Papers* sequence, the voices of the three speakers are
distinguished typographically:

Daughter
Adoptive Mother
Birth Mother

PART I 1961 - 62

Chapter 3: The Waiting Lists

The first agency we went to
didn't want us on their lists,
we didn't live close enough to a church
nor were we church-goers
(though we kept quiet about being communists).
The second told us
we weren't high enough earners.
The third liked us
but they had a five-year waiting list.
I spent six months trying not to look
at swings or the front of supermarket trolleys,
not to think this kid I've wanted could be five.
The fourth agency was full up.
The fifth said yes but again no babies.
Just as we were going out the door
I said oh you know we don't mind the colour.
Just like that, the waiting was over.

This morning a slim manilla envelope arrives
postmarked Edinburgh: one piece of paper
I have now been able to look up your microfiche
(as this is all the records kept nowadays).
From your mother's letters, the following information:
Your mother was nineteen when she had you.
You weighed eight pounds four ounces.
She liked hockey. She worked in Aberdeen
as a waitress. She was five foot eight inches.

I thought I'd hid everything
that there wasnie wan
giveaway sign left

I put Marx Engels Lenin (no Trotsky)
in the airing cupboard—she'll no be
checking out the towels surely
All the copies of the Daily Worker
I shoved under the sofa
the dove of peace I took down from the loo

A poster of Paul Robeson
saying give him his passport
I took down from the kitchen

I left a bust of Burns
my detective stories
and the Complete Works of Shelley

She comes at 11:30 exactly.
I pour her coffee
from my new Hungarian set

And foolishly pray she willnae
ask its origins—honestly
this baby is going to my head.

She crosses her legs on the sofa
I fancy I hear the *Daily Workers*
rustle underneath her

Well she says, you have an interesting home
She sees my eyebrows rise.

190

It's different she qualifies.

Hell and I've spent all morning
trying to look ordinary
—a lovely home for the baby.

She buttons her coat all smiles
I'm thinking
I'm on the home run

But just as we get to the last post
her eye catches at the same times as mine
a red ribbon with twenty world peace badges
Clear as a hammer and sickle
on the wall.
Oh, she says are you against nuclear weapons?

To Hell with this. Baby or no baby.
Yes I says. Yes Yes Yes.
I'd like this baby to live in a nuclear free world.

Oh. Her eyes light up.
I'm all for peace myself she says,
and sits down for another cup of coffee.

Part II 1967 - 1979

Chapter 7: Black Bottom

Maybe that's why I don't like
all this talk about her being black,
I brought her up as my own
as I would any other child
colour matters to the nutters;
but she says my daughter says
it matters to her

I suppose there would have been things
I couldn't understand with any child,
we knew she was coloured.

They told us they had no babies at first
and I chanced it didn't matter what colour it was
and they said *oh well are you sure*
in that case we have a baby for you—
to think she wasn't even thought of as a baby,
my baby, my baby

I chase his *Sambo Sambo* all the way from the school gate.
A fistful of anorak—What did you call me? Say that again.
Sam-bo. He plays the word like a bouncing ball
but his eyes move fast as ping pong.
I shove him up against the wall,
say that again you wee shite. *Sambo, sambo,* he's crying now

I knee him in the balls. What was that?
My fist is steel; I punch and punch his gut.
Sorry I didn't hear you? His tears drip like wax.
Nothing he heaves *I didn't say nothing.*
I let him go. He is a rat running. He turns
and shouts *Dirty Darkie* I chase him again.
Blonde hairs in my hand. Excuse me!
This teacher from primary 7 stops us.
Names? I'll report you to the headmaster tomorrow.
But Miss, Save it for Mr Thompson she says

My teacher's face cracks into a thin smile
Her long nails scratch the note well well
I see you were fighting yesterday, again.
In a few years time you'll be a juvenile delinquent.
Do you know what that is? Look it up in the dictionary.
She spells each letter with slow pleasure.
Read it out to the class.
Thug. Vandal. Hooligan. Speak up. Have you lost your tongue?

To be honest I hardly ever think about it
except if something happens, you know
daft talk about darkies. Racialism.
Mothers ringing my bell with their kids
crying *You tell. You tell. You tell.*
—No. You tell your little girl to stop calling
my little girl names and I'll tell my little girl

to stop giving your little girl a doing.

We're practising for the school show
I'm trying to do the Cha Cha and the Black Bottom
but I can't get the steps right
my right foot's left and my left foot's right
my teacher shouts from the bottom
of the class Come on, show

us what you can do I thought
you people had it in your blood.
My skin is hot as burning coal
like that time she said Darkies are like coal
in front of the whole class—my blood
what does she mean? I thought

she'd stopped all that after the last time
my dad talked to her on parents' night
the other kids are all right till she starts;
my feet step out of time, my heart starts
to miss beats like when I can't sleep at night—
What Is In My Blood? The bell rings, it is time.

**Sometimes it is hard to know what to say
that will comfort. Us two in the armchair;
me holding her breath, "they're ignorant
let's have some tea and cake, forget them."**

Maybe it's really Bette Davis I want
to be the good twin or even better the bad
one or a nanny who drowns a baby in a bath.
I'm not sure maybe I'd prefer Katharine
Hepburn tossing my red hair, having a hot
temper. I says to my teacher Can't I be
Elizabeth Taylor, drunk and fat and she
just laughed, not much chance of that.
I went for an audition for *The Prime
of Miss Jean Brodie*. I didn't get a part
even though I've been acting longer
than Beverley Innes. So I have. Honest.

Olubayo was the colour of peat
when we walked out heads turned
like horses, folk stood like trees
their eyes fixed on us—it made me
burn, that hot glare; my hand
would sweat down to his bone.
Finally, alone, we'd melt
nothing, nothing would matter
He never saw her. I looked for him in her;
for a second it was as if he was there
in that glass cot looking back through her.

On my bedroom wall is a big poster
of Angela Davis who is in prison
right now for nothing at all
except she wouldn't put up with stuff.
My mum says she is *only* 26
which seems really old to me
but my mum says it is young

just imagine, she says, being on
America's Ten Most Wanted People's List at 26!
I can't.
Angela Davis is the only female person
I've seen (except for a nurse on TV)
who looks like me. She had big hair like mine
that grows out instead of down.
My mum says it's called an *Afro*.
If I could be as brave as her when I get older
I'll be OK.
Last night I kissed her goodnight again
and wondered if she could feel the kisses
in prison all the way from Scotland.
Her skin is the same too you know.
I can see my skin is that colour
but most of the time I forget,
so sometimes when I look in the mirror
I give myself a bit of a shock
and say to myself *Do you really look like this?*
as if I'm somebody else. I wonder if she does that.

I don't believe she killed anybody.
It is all a load of phoney lies.
My dad says it's a set up.
I asked him if she'll get the electric chair
like them Roseberries he was telling me about.
No he says the world is on her side.
Well how come she's in there then I thinks.
I worry she's going to get the chair.
I worry she's worrying about the chair.
My dad says she'll be putting on a brave face.
He brought me a badge home which I wore
to school. It says FREE ANGELA DAVIS.
And all my pals says "Who's she?"

PART III 1980 - 1990

Chapter 8: Generations

The sun went out just like that
almost as if it had never been,
hard to imagine now the way it fell
on treetops, thatched roofs, people's faces.
Suddenly the trees lost their nerves
and the grass passed the wind on
blade to blade, fast as gossip

Years later, the voices still come close
especially in dreams, not distant echoes
loud—a pneumatic drill—deeper and deeper still.
I lived the scandal, wore it casual
as a summer's dress, Jesus sandals.
All but the softest whisper:
she's lost an awful lot of weight.

Now my secret is the hush of heavy curtains drawn.
I dread strange handwriting
sometimes jump when the phone rings,
she is all of nineteen and legally able.

At night I lie practising my lines
but "sorry" never seems large enough
nor "I can't see you, yes, I'll send a photograph."

I was pulled out with forceps
left a gash down my left cheek
four months inside a glass cot
but
she came faithful from Glasgow to Edinburgh
and peered through the glass
she would not pick another baby.

I don't know what diseases
come down my line;
when dentist and doctors ask
the old blood questions about family runnings
I tell them: I have no nose or mouth or eyes
to match, no spitting image or dead cert,
my face watches itself in the glass.

I have my parents who are not of the same tree
and you keep trying to make it matter,
the blood, the tie, the passing down
generations.
We all have our contradictions,
the ones with the mother's nose and father's eyes
have them;
the blood does not bind confusion,
yet I confess to my contradiction
I want to know my blood.

I know my blood.
It is dark ruby red and comes
regular and I use Lillets.
I know my blood when I cut my finger.
I know what my blood looks like.

It is the well, the womb, the fucking seed.
Here, I am far enough away to wonder—
what were their faces like
who were my grandmothers
what were the days like

passed in Scotland
the land I come from
the soil in my blood.

Put it this way:
I know she thinks of me often
when the light shows its face
or the dark skulks behind hills,
she conjures me up or I just appear
when I take the notion, my slippers
are silent and I walk through doors.

She's lying in bed; I wake her up
a pinch on her cheek is enough,
then I make her think of me for hours.
The best thing I can steal is sleep.
I get right under the duvet and murmur
you'll never really know your mother.
I know who she thinks I am—she's made a blunder.

She is faceless
She has no nose
She is five foot eight inches tall
She likes hockey best
She is twenty-six today
She was a waitress
My hair is grey
She wears no particular dress
The skin around my neck is wrinkling
Does she imagine me this way?
Lately I make pictures of her
But I can see the smallness
She is tall and slim
of her hands, Yes
Her hair is loose curls
an opal stone on her middle finger
I reach out to catch her
Does she talk broad Glasgow?
But no matter how fast
Maybe they moved years ago
I run after

She is faceless, she never
weeps. She has neither eyes nor
fine boned cheeks

Once would be enough,
just to listen to her voice
watch the way she moves her hands
when she talks.

SHAY YOUNGBLOOD

Did My Mama Like to Dance?

Grown folks could be so mysterious bout certain things. Big Mama, Aunt Mae and Aunt Viola would bend my ears back bout obeying God and my elders, talk bout everybody—only in the most Christian way, of course—and everything cept my blood mama, Fannie Mae. One time I heard somebody say she died from dancing. Somebody else I heard say she died from an old wound that was too deep to heal. I was getting to be twelve and real curious bout her.

I used to not care much bout her, hardly thought bout her cept on Mother's Day when Big Mama took me and Brother to the cemetery to put flowers on her grave. I thought bout her the time I was at Jan's birthday party when Gwen Jackson told me I had no business pointing my finger cause my mama was dead. Her words give me a hurting in my heart that was worse than a belt lick on my behind. The sweet piece of chocolate cake Miss Louise cut for me tasted like dry dumplings in my throat, and my crying stained the pretty pink tablecloth. I got up from that kitchen table and run home to Big Mama who set the table for a party just for me and her.

There was a few pictures of Fannie Mae round, but the only way I could picture her was asleep at her funeral. It seemed like a dream. I was bout six the day that Brother bust in the room I shared with Big Mama, all out of breath. I was laying across the big double bed, reading a comic book.

"Fannie Mae dead," he said, looking hurt and lost.

I almost asked him who he was talking bout before I said, "Oh." The only other thing I could think to say was, "That mean we can't go up north, now?"

Brother fell on his knees and started crying.

"Please don't cry, Brother," I begged him. His crying scared me. He was older and stronger than me, and even when he got beat for doing something bad, like cussing in church, I never saw him cry. I guess he remembered Fannie Mae better than me.

At the funeral a few days later I remember sitting in the last pew in the church with Miss Corine, the beautician, on one side of me, and big, fat Aunt Viola on the other. Brother was too broke up to come. That was the first time he run away from home. The church was full. People was standing in the back of the church when chairs and pews ran out. It was hot, and there wasn't a breeze nowhere, though a whole lot of Pitts Funeral Home fans was waving hot air round. A soldierly row of lady ushers in white dresses, shoes, stockings and white lace hankies on they heads stood in the middle aisle humming with one white-gloved hand resting over they hearts. The two male ushers was dressed in black suits. They white gloves looked like they was separated from they bodies.

The singing coming from the choir stand that day was sad. I could hear people up in the front crying and hollering. I remember being fascinated by the peculiar shine on my new black patent leather shoes and the lace ruffle on my new socks. The heat made me sleepy, so I edged up close to Aunt Vi and leaned into her softness and slept peacefully for a while. Somebody shook me awake out of a nice dream. Aunt Vi took my hand, and we started walking out of the pew. I thought we was leaving, but we was headed for the front of the church. When we got there Aunt Vi picked me up and held me over the long white casket surrounded by flowers and standing wreaths. Fannie Mae lay inside looking like she had fall asleep. She was so beautiful it made my throat hurt to look at her.

"Do you know who this is?" Aunt Vi asked me.

"It's Fannie Mae, ain't it?" I whispered.

"She's in the Lord's hands now," Aunt Vi whispered back. "We don't have to worry bout her being too pretty no more. She through dancing now."

When I was a lil older and wanted someone to remember my mama to me, all the begging I could manage wouldn't move Big Mama, Aunt Vi or Aunt Mae to talk much bout her. Every time I asked Big Mama, she would look off somewhere over my shoulder and get real misty-eyed.

"She was a beautiful chile. Cut down just as she was starting to grow. You just like her. Look like she spit you outta her mouth." Then she wouldn't say nothing for a while. Even though I would sit quiet waiting for her to go on she never would.

When I asked Aunt Mae, who told me most everything else I wanted to know, she would almost get tongue-tied and start to cry or reach for a glass of whiskey to calm her down.

"Don't start me to crying, baby. Your mama is dead and buried, don't raise her up to haint me. Some things just ain't meant to be said out loud once they passed."

Aunt Vi would start to rocking back and forth and humming when I asked her. I decided that I needed to talk to someone outside the family. If anybody would know bout Fannie Mae's mystery and tell me, it was gonna be Miss Corine. She knew everybody's business. Cause she ran the beauty shop on Front Street, she was in a position to listen in on everybody's life—first, second and third-hand. She was also in a position to give her opinion on a lot of things. Standing over somebody's head for two or more hours gains they full attention.

Miss Corine was nearly six feet tall, and she'd tell anybody quick she had pure Indian blood in her. Seminole. Her mama's people was from Florida. Some of them still lived on a reservation. You could look at her red-brown skin and the long, black braid that hung down her back, high cheekbones and clear brown eyes that slanted upward at the corners and see that. She was also quick to admit to South Carolina Geechee on her daddy's side, which is why some folks said she talked funny, ate so much rice, and the reason her fingers could braid the wind. On top of looking good, Miss Corine could put a hot curl in the shortest, nappiest of naps and untangle thick, sassy hair on a tender-headed chile without a single tear. Some called her a miracle worker.

For me, going to Miss Corine's shop first thing on a Saturday morning was better than a birthday present. Usually I hung round the shop hours after she finished with my head, helping out. I would straighten up the stacks of magazines, empty ashtrays and collect the balls of hair that fell from ladies' heads over the course of the morning and afternoon sessions. I would collect the hair in a paper sack for later when Miss Corine would help me make braids and wigs for my dolls who all had the wrong kinda hair—all straight and obedient. At least they skin was brown like mine. Mostly though, I sat listening to Miss Corine and the other customers who Big Mama called the walking-talking-newspapers.

Miss Corine's shop was situated in a small storefront, in between Pitts Funeral Home and Fat Daddy's Rib Shack. *Miss Corine's Beauty Shop* was painted in beautiful red-and-white script on the plate glass window of the shop. A crooked hand-lettered cardboard sign was stuck in the lower left-hand corner of the window. It read: *We Curl Up & Dye*.

It was a three-chair shop built shotgun-style, long and narrow. The walls and ceiling were painted a bright pink, and the floor was covered in black-and-white squares of linoleum. One long wall was lined with six, low, red vinyl stuffed chairs with heavy chrome armrests. A couple of low tables were stacked high with outdated hair and fashion magazines, as well as *Black True Romance* and some comic books. A small black-and-white TV was kept on during business hours. It sat on a table in the front window surrounded by Miss Corine's plants. There was a mirror running the length of the other wall and a ledge underneath it where beauty and hair supplies were kept. Three black leather styling chairs that swiveled and raised to the expert touch of Miss Corine were welded into the floor.

At the back of the shop there was a big red-and-white Coke machine, and on the right was the door to the ladies room, a tiny place with a one-seater and a cracked mirror above a pink porcelain sink and another stack of magazines. A small window on the wall at the back of the shop looked on an alley that faced a red brick wall. Miss Corine had pretty pink curtains on that window. The screen door at the other end of the shop kept flies out in the summertime and invited callers year round. The shop door was always open and somebody was usually hollering in at Miss Corine.

Once inside the shop the strong scent of Sulphur 8 hair grease was like a salve to my soul. I knew I wasn't far from a good feeling. Miss Mary said Miss Corine should've been a healer cause when she laid her hands on your head you were healed of whatever laid heavy on your heart and mind. Nobody could hardly keep from telling her what was on they mind.

Big Mama sent me to Miss Corine's every second Saturday to get my hair washed, conditioned and straightened out. Big Mama said she almost cry when she have to do my hair for school every morning, it be so thick and woolly. Said she was getting too old to tangle with my naps. This one particular Saturday I had made up my mind to ask Miss Corine bout my mama, no matter the consequence or reaction. I waited till Miss Corine had me sitting in the low-back leather chair, my head leaned back in the wash sink, under the pressure of warm water, and Miss Corine's deep massaging fingers on my scalp.

"Miss Corine, how long you know my blood mama?" I asked, knowing the worst she could do was not answer me like Big Mama. But Miss Corine don't hardly hold back nothing.

"Chile, I knowed your mama before she was knee-high to a duck. She worked here in this shop for two years."

"What was she like Miss Corine?"

"Ain't your Big Mama tell you bout her?"

"No m'am, not much. They say it hurt too much to talk bout her. Sometime Aunt Mae call me by her name and start to cry."

"She right. You look just like your mama. Fannie Mae was a real pretty

girl, and nice too. Even though she was high yellow she didn't have no attitude. Always had her nose in a fashion magazine. If she said it once, she said
it a thousand times: 'Miss Corine, I'm going to New York and wear dresses
like that and when I do my dance everybody gonna scream.' When Carlos
come through here headed north, I could see the writing on the wall . . ."

She paused a minute, then asked me, "What you want to know, baby?"

"Did my mama like to dance?"

Miss Corine didn't say nothing. She finished rinsing my hair, then wrapped
my naps in a thick, white towel and led me to the styling chair. I was just bout
to repeat myself when Miss Lamama, dressed in a long, orange tie-dyed dress,
opened the screen door and stuck her turban-wrapped head in.

"Corine, Rosa want to know if she can borrow one of your curling irons.
She dropped hers on the concrete floor and they broke in two. She's working
on Sister Davis next door."

"Sister Davis had a stroke didn't she? The pressure of all them crazy children of hers finally sent her to an early grave."

"Yes, my dear. The good sister died in her sleep, and she wasn't but fifty-
seven years old."

"I know Rosa will do her head justice. Give her these. She can have em,
they a spare."

I was thinking that Miss Rosa probably curled my mama's hair when she
died. I'd have to thank her one day cause Fannie Mae looked pretty good.
When Miss Lamama left with the curling iron, Miss Corine took up where
she left off on my head and started to talk bout Fannie Mae without me
pushing.

"Your mama was consumed by love. Love is what took her away from us."

"What you mean?"

"She loved dancing too strong, and that chile loved the truth. When she
and Carlos left here all Fannie Mae could see was a way to dance. I was in
love with something once so I knowed what it look like."

"Was she good?"

"At dancing? Hmph! She was better than good at most things she did, but
that didn't have nothing to do with it. You ever look out the back window at
that brick wall across the lot?"

"Yes m'am."

"Well, that brick wall is just as hard as your mama's head was then. She was
stubborn. She kept forgetting she was a colored woman living in the deep
and backward South, and that it was 1956. It was before integration, before
equal opportunities, before civil rights demonstrations was all on the TV
and in the newspapers."

"What happened in 1956?" I egged her on, excited to find out anything bout Fannie Mae.

"What happened! How old you is chile?"

"I'm almost twelve," I said, like almost twelve was grown enough to know whatever she was getting ready to say.

"Then you old enough to know what happened. Fannie Mae was thirteen when she got in trouble the first time. Wasn't her fault either. She got picked up for talking back to a white man. She was buying some things from the grocery store and the storekeeper was trying to cheat her. Now your mama knew her numbers. She wasn't nobody's fool. She knew how to figure, so she called him a liar. He hauled off and slapped her down. Then he had the gall to call the police on her. They took her down to juvenile detention. Chile, it wasn't no fence high enough to keep Fannie Mae where she didn't wanna be. She broke out of that place and hitched a ride to New Orleans. But they caught her and drug her back in a week or two.

"Now your mama's pride was her long pretty hair, a good grade and thick, too. She used to wrap it on top of her head like a crown. When she fixed up you'd swear she was a movie star. When they brought her back the last time, them animals cut all her hair off. Yes m'am, they shaved that poor chile's head clean. Not to be held back, she found a way out again and hooked up with a soldier. They married over in Alabama. That was a joke. Your mama just wanted a way out of that stinking jail. On her honeymoon night she said she made that boy sleep on the porch of his mama's house. She run away from him too. Come back to live with your Aunt Mae. Then trouble seemed to run after her."

Miss Corine kept parting my hair and lathering each gap with Sulphur 8, soothing the tension out of her words. She stopped for a minute to blow her nose and wipe the sweat out of her eyes.

"Baby, I understand why your Big Mama and your aunties ain't told you bout her. The telling hurts. It bring up too many memories. You getting to be a woman now, and God knows you need to hear this. Hold still now. I'm getting ready to put the hot comb to your head."

I held my head down, chin to chest, waiting for the sizzle of hot metal comb on damp, greased naps. Miss Corine's hands were steady, never jerking or burning the tender skin on my neck.

While I was waiting for Miss Corine to get to the next chapter in Fannie Mae's story, Mr. Pitts from the funeral home next door hollered in the door. "What you know good, Corine?"

"Couldn't be better, Pitts. How's business?" Miss Corine hollered back at him.

"Dead as ever," he said, laughing at his own joke.

Big Mama said Mr. Pitts could make a dead man laugh, she said he could make you forget you was mourning somebody. He buried Fannie Mae. I heard folks say he was in love with her. As if she read my mind, when Mr. Pitts left Miss Corine say, "Pitts used to take your mama to the picture show. Buy her all the candy and popcorn she could hold. He really loved your mama like she was his chile. She made him laugh. Where a lot of mens would've taken advantage of a pretty young girl like Fannie Mae, he showed her nothing but kindness and respect, and she give him the same. When she was a lil girl, she was here in my shop messing round or over in the funeral home arranging flowers for Mr. Pitts and Miss Rosa."

There was a quiet space where I spoke my heart.

"I used to hate Fannie Mae," I confessed for the first time to anybody. "I hated her for leaving me and then for being dead. One time I locked myself in the bathroom cause I didn't want to wear no white flower on my new white dress on Mother's Day, letting everybody know my mama was dead. I cried so hard Big Mama felt bad for me. I ended up wearing a red and white flower. Big Mama convinced me how important it was to respect the dead as well as the living."

"I remember that. You almost broke your Big Mama's heart. She knew then how strong you felt bout losing your mama and she felt so helpless, wasn't nothing she could do then."

There was a light tapping on the door and Miss Rosa came in. She was tiny and elegant, like her brother Mr. Pitts. She always wore a hat to match her dress. I wondered if she slept in them hats. Her delicate smile was warm, and her light green eyes invited your confidence and trust. She stepped into the shop gently and looked round for attention like she was bout to make an announcement.

"Corine, on behalf of myself and Mr. Pitts I would like to thank you for the use of your curling irons," Miss Rosa said.

"You been working on Sister Davis, Jessie say."

"Sister Davis was a good Christian woman, a nice-looking woman, but she aged so quickly. All those children I suppose. At any rate, I thank you for your generosity."

"Rosa, you know you welcome to them old irons and anything else I have. When is Sister Davis' funeral?"

"Tomorrow morning, and I do not look forward to dealing with her heathen children. They chose the cheapest casket and arrangements for the dear woman, and I know for a fact that her insurance policy would have more than covered a decent burial." Miss Rosa coughed a delicate cough, then cleared her throat a few times. I took my chance to thank her.

"Miss Rosa, I don't remember my mama very much, but I remember how pretty you made her look for the funeral. Thank you for making her look so nice."

"Why thank you, chile," she said, as if seeing me for the first time. "You look so much like her. She was a lovely girl, so smart and talented. We all loved her. Her passing was a great loss. In all my days I never seen so many grown men cry at a funeral. Mr. Pitts wept the whole time he worked on her. He sent her the money to come home, but she never made it. Didn't she love to dance, Jesus!"

Miss Rosa sniffed and wiped her teary eyes on a black lace hanky she had tied to her wrist.

"She really loved you. She wanted you to be with her. I believe she's much happier with the Lord."

Miss Rosa stood there staring at me for a few minutes, then tossed up her hanky and stepped out the door.

"Everybody loved your mama," Miss Corine went on with her story. "Like I said, she was a good girl, but trouble seemed to follow her."

"What kind of trouble?" I asked, a lil scared of what I might hear.

"When your mama turned fifteen, she got a scholarship to a lil integrated dance school downtown. First of its kind. Run by some crazy white ladies from up north. Fannie Mae and this white girl—Patty, I think her name was—got to be good friends. One day Patty and your mama was holding hands walking in the white folks' park. Fannie Mae forgot all bout them signs and things. She and Patty got to laughing and dancing down the street and over the grass them white folks claimed was theirs. Fannie Mae was so pretty. Too pretty. Some white boys noticed them and asked Patty what she was doing holding hands with a nigger. Before they could run or holler or anything, them boys raped them both. Raped them in that lil park down on Main Street in broad daylight. Scarred them girls up for life. Policeman's son."

I was hurting when she said that. My throat tightened up, but I held back the tears. I'd come too far to turn round. "Aunt Mae say all the time, 'Mama's baby, Poppa's maybe,'" I say. "I just want to know bout Fannie Mae."

Miss Corine looked at me in a sad, knowing way and kept on talking.

"There was a big trial, and if the lawyer hadn't a been so scared of that policeman's weight, your mama would've won. She bent after that. But you know she was more determined than ever to keep dancing. She worked out every night after she helped me here in this shop. She was still a chile at fifteen when you was born. Your Big Mama fell in love with you and took to keeping you more than your mama. After a while Fannie Mae felt like she couldn't claim y'all no more. All she had was love, and that don't feed hungry children. She left here and went up north. She found a job cleaning up in a dance hall. Your Big Mama and Aunt Mae felt like it was they fault she died on that dance floor, fell out from a brain tumor, washing away her dreams. Dreams die hard. Some say her spirit broke."

Miss Corine paused with the hot comb in mid-air. I could see her reflection in the mirror, proud chin set tight, eyes trying not to cry. I couldn't hold back no more. I cried till my eyes hurt, till my heart was empty and my soul full. I whispered thanks into the front of Miss Corine's pink uniform, for the pain she had to bear to tell me the truth. She held me close, stroking my hair and rocking me back and forth.

"Now that's all I know, baby. It wasn't all a pretty picture, but it's the one I seen."

Miss Corine wiped my tears and gave me a tissue to blow my nose in. Her rich hands caressed my back and eased the pain that truth could bring.

"If you don't remember nothing else I tell you baby, you remember this: If you got to dance or dream or anything at all, take it a step at a time and don't let nothing and nobody get in your way when you doing right. I ain't saying it's gonna be easy, but we all got a dance to do. You remember this, you hear?"

"Yes m'am," I answered, still wiping away my tears.

They Tell Me . . . Now I Know

When I was a lil girl I knew the day was coming when I would join the circle of women. I knew cause Big Mama told me, and so did Aunt Mae every time I asked bout the lives of grown folks, or the sounds I heard behind late-night doors. Love, sex and money. Grown folks' business. I waited for the day with the same longing as birthdays and Christmas because presents were promised as well as secrets and answers to questions only a grownup could know. I knew the day I became a woman would be marked by blood.

The summer I turned twelve I got my first sign. Soon all the women in the community knew. Big Mama announced it at a regular meeting of the #2 Mission Prayer Circle as new business.

"Daughter got her blood this morning!" I heard Big Mama say. "We gonna have to take her to the river."

"I could've told you that. I seen the signs, I had the dream," Miss Mary put in.

"Look like time done sneaked up on us. She's becoming a woman. We gotta keep a sharp eye on her," Aunt Mae winked at Miss Corine. "The boys'll be sniffing round her like hound dogs afterwhile."

"By the time her mama come to us she was already on the road to ruin. It was too late to take her to the river . . ."

"Too late to take her anywhere. She was too fast . . ."

"And too pretty. Somebody had done already whispered something in her ear. She come in the door dancing."

"Left dancing, too. She left this world dreaming just like she come in."

"We can give Daughter what we couldn't give her mama."

"Daughter been restless, asking lotta questions."

"Bout time she got some answers."

"Her gifts, too."

"Yeah, we can give Daughter what we couldn't give Fannie Mae."

After the meeting broke up I was called into the room and all the women hugged me good-night. I went upstairs to get ready for bed. Big Mama stayed up to wash the tea glasses and serving plates and read some from her Bible. Suddenly I was scared. They had mentioned the river. Snakes, prickly briars and drowning. I had so many questions, thoughts and feelings. I was still wide awake when Big Mama walked softly into the bedroom. I watched her undress in the dark and pull her worn flannel nightgown over her head.

"Big Mama?"

"I didn't mean to wake you up, baby."

"I couldn't go to sleep, Big Mama. When y'all gonna take me to the river?"

"On your birthday. We got all summer long to get you ready."

"Why I have to go now? I don't wanna go."

"Baby, your blood's come. There's some things you need to know and going to the river is a thing you need to do."

"It's a long way to the river."

She laughed, "Don't have to be no river there."

"Well, what happens at the river?"

"When a girlchile get her first blood her mama or one like her mama have to prepare her. Tell her things a woman needs to know. Then the women in the family can take her to a secret place for the crossing over."

Big Mama held my hand and started humming what sounded like one of Miss Lamama's African songs, whispering words I didn't understand. I felt comforted by the darkness. The song and the music drifted into my dreams of forests dripping with fine sprays of blood instead of rain.

I started spending more time alone with my Big Mamas. I kept hoping for presents like a camera, new clothes or jewelry on my visits. Instead they gave me stories.

Aunt Mae's way of getting me ready was to explain human desires. "You feel like you wanna kiss somebody and hug em, that's alright. Nothing wrong with showing affection."

"What if they wanna have sex, Aunt Mae?"

"Now, Daughter, you just twelve years old and I'm over sixty, so I've lived long enough to know sex ain't all it's made out to be. If you love somebody you can both wait till you ready to be responsible bout having sex. In the meantime you gonna have feelings, desire for being close to somebody. I'm gonna tell you like my mama told me. If it gets hot, fan it. If you cain't wait, stop long enough to make him wear a rubber. Look like we gonna have to make a trip to the health department and don't you tell sister, she'll just have a fit. You wanna hear bout the first time I made love with a man?"

"Yeah, Aunt Mae."

"Reverend Isaiah Masterson was his name. Oh, now he wasn't a reverend when I met him. The only thing holy bout Isaiah then was his name. That man was smooth as glass. Move me like Mahalia's singing, and he was sweet as Karo syrup. Met him at a house party on Cornbread Row. My girlfriend Peaches saw him first, but it was me he asked to dance. He took me round that dance floor like I was a mop. I was weak with desire and I didn't know exactly what it was. He blew in my ear, told me I was pretty and sweet-talked me into one of the back bedrooms. I was out of my clothes so fast he must've thought I was a professional. I was twenty years old and still living at home with my mama. I'd been thinking bout it and listening to my girlfriends go on bout it and I knew he was the one.

"Especially when he asked me if I was using any protection. I hadn't even thought bout that. Then I got scared. The last thing I wanted was to get pregnant at that time. Well, fortunately he was prepared. When I told him I was a virgin, he laughed so loud I thought somebody was gonna come in. He was gentle, such a sweet man. It hurt like the devil, and there was a lil blood.

"When he was finished that sweet man turned over and slept like somebody hit him over the head. I knew that wasn't gonna do. I woke him up after awhile and told him he forgot something. I asked him wasn't I sposed to feel something. He look all embarrassed, then asked me what I wanted. I told him I didn't know, but he hadn't got to it yet. He laughed again like he did when I told him I was a virgin. Said I didn't sound like a virgin. I told him not to mistake me for a fool. Never had so much fun in my life after that.

Now that was an experienced man, just a lil lazy. He ain't had but one rubber so he had to get real creative. Never met another man quite like him.

"But there's more to being together than making love, and Isaiah moved round too much. Here today gone tomorrow. Chile, don't get involved with a travelin man unless you wanna spend a lotta time looking out the window waiting for trains and crying."

Miss Mary, Miss Tom, Miss Lamama and the other women told me bout some more things I'd need to know to get on in the white man's world, as they called it.

"Keep your own money—be independent."

"Treat other folks like you wanna be treated, but let no one walk over you. Stand up for yourself."

"Remember where you come from. You meet the same folks on the way up as you do on the way down."

"Pray. Put faith in the Lord and in yourself."

"If you don't want a baby, keep your legs crossed and your dress tail down."

"Let not your heart be troubled, the Lord is watching over you."

My thirteenth birthday was on a Saturday in late September. It was a beautiful, crisp day. Everything was clear, sharp. Downstairs Big Mama was cooking my favorite breakfast—pancakes, fried oysters and meal-fried green tomatoes. A bunch of wild flowers and a basket of fruit were on the coffee table, with a pink birthday card signed by all my Big Mamas.

When night come, so did the women. Me, Big Mama and Miss Corine got into Aunt Mae's big white fishtail Cadillac. The other women rode with Miss Lamama, who was driving her husband's taxicab. We ended up at our church. Miss Lamama had a key since she was head of the Usher Board. It was strange being there with just the eight of us in the red-carpeted, softly lit room.

Big Mama took me into the pastor's study and dressed me in a snow white choir robe and tied my hair with a length of white gauzy material. She kissed me and led me back into the church where the other women had changed into different rainbow-colored robes. Miss Lamama wore yellow, Miss Corine wore pink, Miss Mary wore purple, Aunt Mae wore red. Big Mama put on a royal blue robe. Aunt Vi wore a lavender one, and Miss Tom wore green. It was dark, and each woman carried a short, fat white candle that smelled of vanilla and a small bundle wrapped in white cloth. They gathered round me as we headed out the back door. In the quiet clearing between the tall pines I could smell the pine sap and feel the soft pine needles under my bare feet.

The women circled me and began to sing Miss Lamama's African song. *Yemenjah, Yemenjah. . . .* Miss Mary beat her drum, and Miss Lamama shook her prized red-beaded calabash.

Big Mama entered the circle and faced me. She spoke first. "That your eyes may see truth and heart have faith in things you cannot see." She dipped her finger in a small wooden bowl and touched my forehead and chest with oil.

"That your arms and hands find productive work, that is helpful to your neighbor." Miss Mary touched my shoulders and hands with the oil, which had been passed to her.

"That your feet carry you away and back to us when it is time," Miss Corine said.

"May you love with your heart and eyes wide open," Miss Tom said.

"Welcome, Rita, never fear, we are with you always near. Close to the river, moon bleed through . . ."

"We will guide you, guide you through," all the women responded.

Each woman called me by my name as they gave me my gift, hugging me, their tears mingling with mine. Big Mama gave me a small Bible with a white-beaded cover I knew had belonged to her mother. Miss Mary placed some of her special protection beads round my neck. Miss Corine laid a beautiful silk scarf over my head. Miss Lamama laid a length of heavy African cloth over my left shoulder and kissed me on both cheeks. Aunt Mae put a handful of five-dollar bills into a small change purse attached to a string and placed it round my neck. Aunt Vi sprayed me with my first perfume from a cut-glass atomizer bottle. Miss Tom gave me a book of poems by Langston Hughes.

I felt a cool breeze. It must've been the strong incense and the brightness of the candles that caused me to see my blood mama, Fannie Mae, standing behind the trees blowing me a kiss. She seemed to float away in my memory. These women were my mamas. They had always been there to give me whatever I thought I needed. Standing in that circle of light behind the Eighth Street Baptist Church on a clear September night I was given my name and invited into the circle of women, no longer a lil girl. I was a woman now. All the stories they had told me were gifts, all the love more precious than gold. They tell me . . . now I know.

SUSAN MISAO DAVIE

An Adoptee's Journal

My story is about birth and adoption. I was born to a Japanese mother and a Caucasian father and given up for adoption. Although my physical appearance strongly favors my Asian heritage, three years ago I gave birth to a blond-haired, blue-eyed baby girl. Her birth stirred up some ancient dust from my own birth. Her blue eyes propelled me into a dark journey.

February 1991   I did not see or feel my baby's birth. I had a baby, yet because she was born by Caesarean section, the connection I'd been waiting for was not there. I loved her, but was she really mine? She didn't look like me. Maybe she had gotten mixed up with another baby in the nursery, and I'd never know if I had the right one. When I brought her home, I said, "You're adopted." I was playing with the words. I couldn't believe my birth mother had given away a baby that small and defenseless. I couldn't imagine letting someone else have her. Who could love her as much as I did? A baby needs its own mother.

Of course I knew she was my baby. But I lost the thing I wanted most in life, which was to feel what it was like to be blood-related to someone. Having a baby was the only way I'd ever get a blood relative. I hadn't wanted her to be out of my sight after she was born—so I'd be sure she wouldn't get lost, stolen, mixed up or given away—but she spent her first night away from me. In fact, she was rarely with me for the four days I was in the hospital. Why did that make me feel like she wasn't mine? It was me, losing my mother all over again. Even her name, Alyce, had been my own birth name.

April 13   Yesterday I got the "non-identifying" information I had requested over a year ago. It said my birth mother's labor was uncomplicated and only five hours long. I wish I had known that before Alyce's birth. And my father was a Russian Jew! Also he had blond hair and blue eyes.

July 30 I thought having a baby would make up for not having "parents." It doesn't, but I like the baby. I think losing your baby would be worse than losing your mother.

August 6 I called this search person, and she found my birth mother! It was so fast. I told her my original last name, and she typed it into her computer and said, "Alyce?" Oh, my God. I said yes, and she told me my birth mother's maiden name. Then her new name, address and phone number. I actually tried to call, but no one answered. That's probably a good thing. All these years of wondering, and with just a few phone calls I find out where she is. I'm so glad she's not dead. I hope she wants to meet me. I wrote her a letter and asked her to call or write me, and I sent her a picture of me and Alyce.

I hope I hope I hope I get to meet my birth mom.

August 7 The mailman came and took my letter to my birth mother today. Bill says I should wait two weeks and then call her. I really want her to call or write me, because if two weeks go by and I haven't heard anything, I'll be paranoid she doesn't want to meet me.

August 13 What if she never writes back? How will I know if she ever got my letter? Or if she's really the one? If I don't hear from her, I'll try once more and then give up. At least I'll die knowing I tried.

August 26 I'm in limbo now. People keep asking if I've heard from my birth mother. I wonder if I was smart to share this with so many people.

September 17 I still haven't heard anything. Everything is different now though: I guess because I've been a mother for almost eight months, I'm less preoccupied with the past and more into the future. I still would love to hear from my birth mother and meet her, or have a picture of her, but now it doesn't seem as important. (Or am I just denying its importance since it looks as if nothing will happen?) Finding out her name and address seems to be enough for now.

September 19 I think I searched for my birth mom to complete the scenario: I have a mom, but I'm missing the mom I started out with—I wanted to fill in that part. I'm sad for the baby who was separated from her mom way back then.

October 30 I don't know. This whole adoption thing. I'm kind of depressed about it because it's basically unsolvable: I'm adopted, and that can never change. I thought Alyce would fill the hole inside me, but she didn't. Life with her is all brand new. Even if I met my birth mother, and even if she liked me and wanted to know me, it wouldn't erase my adoption. It's not that adoption is a bad thing necessarily, but you can't get around it. I had a mother, and a father, and the three of us were in some way a "family," though never to be together. Even though I'm somebody, I'm not who I would have been. Being adopted is like free-floating: I have no anchor. My adoptive parents, of course, were my family. But not being their real child permeates my whole life. Now I have to deal with my birth mother, who still hasn't written back. I know I'll try to make contact again. I have no choice. I could pick up the phone and call her, or go down there and try to see her, but I'm afraid.

I think my depression after Alyce's birth had more to do with my adoption than with the Caesarean. Throughout my pregnancy I had this feeling that I wouldn't get to keep my baby.

Finding my birth mother will be satisfying only to a certain point: It could be good, but it will not be best, so I have to prepare myself for that emotionally, because I don't want to get totally messed up. I'm really tired of being messed up, and I really have no choice about it: I have to be messed up the rest of my life. I don't know if I should have another baby, but it seems like I've set myself on this path where I already have one child, why not have another and make it a real family? I'm really into this "family" thing. It's like my whole life begins here. I don't have a history, and Alyce's history will be all wrapped up in Bill's family—I'm still nowhere.

What should I do? Maybe I'll call her. Maybe I should just take a trip down there and try and see her; you know, spy on her, then call her up. If she totally rejects me, I'll feel really bad, and that's what I want to avoid. Living in this limbo is almost preferable.

November 2 What would my life be without Alyce? A lot of things would still be shoved back. Having a baby has pushed me into this whole new world and showed me things about my own self that I had ignored for so long. It's like being reborn. Alyce is discovering life, and I'm discovering it right alongside of her.

November 4 When I look in the mirror, I don't see anything at all. I have no history, no reason for who I am.

November 12 I never realized until I had a child how hard it would be to give your baby away.

November 21 I'm really desperate to contact her, just to know who birthed me.

November 22 I wrote another letter to my birth mother today. I have nothing to lose.

November 27 Today my birth mother called me on the telephone! Imagine that.

It was pretty weird talking to her. I didn't feel as if I was talking to my mother, just talking to a person I really wanted to talk to and was afraid of losing again. I was afraid to ask too much. But I really can't believe she called. It's all I've thought about for the last six hours. I have a birth mother! She's Japanese! I already knew that. I asked her a bunch of questions. I was so nervous, and I think she was, too. She said she didn't think about searching for me but did think about me a lot. She said she destroyed the letters I wrote so her husband wouldn't find them, but saved the pictures I sent of me and Alyce.

She said my birth father did know about me. She wouldn't tell me his name. She said she would if it was an emergency—I don't know what that means, maybe if I needed a bone marrow transplant or something. She said she kept me for a week before giving me up for adoption. She said she has two daughters and a son.

I asked her to send me a picture of herself. I kept thinking of things I wanted to ask, but everything I thought of I'd think, no, I better not ask that, it's too personal; I didn't want to scare her off. We talked for maybe fifteen minutes. I said, "So it's true? You're really the one?" and she said, "Oh, yes."

I am really happy she called me. I just keep wanting more and more.

I feel really connected tonight. Alyce has a Japanese grandmother. I am really happy for her to have that. I feel more a part of this world tonight. I feel connected to the earth. My half brother and sisters have children who are my real nieces and nephews, and I have lots of real aunts and uncles.

November 28 I thought about her again today. I thought of more questions, and I thought about all the things that happened thirty-four years ago.

I tried to imagine what it's like for her to be bringing that all to the surface again. We are two strangers who are thinking about the exact same thing.

November 29 Still thinking about her all the time and wondering what's going to happen. Will she call me again? Should I call her? How long should I wait before I call her? What should I say? What do I want from her? All my life I've been searching for the truth.

December 2 It's been five days since she called, and she hasn't called me back yet! I don't expect her to call for a while, but I might have to call her sometime before Christmas because I just can't stand it.

You can't know what it's like to have this person within my reach, but still not reachable. What if she's ugly? What if she's mean? She's my mother, she has to be nice. When she called and told me who she was, I think I went into shock and didn't talk or sound like me at all. I hate that.

I really want to be related. I guess I'm always trying to know what it's like. Bill looks more like his father every day. His sister does, too, but she has the mannerisms of their mom. It's weird to watch people become more like their parents. I was always glad that no one would ever see me growing to look and act like anyone else, even though I wanted to know who I looked and acted like.

December 3 I thought the way I felt after she called me was the way I was always going to feel, but now it's changing and it's kind of scary because it could get real big in my head and out of my control. What is she thinking of me? I asked her questions and was too nervous to listen to the answers. She asked if I wanted to meet my brother and sisters, and I just stuttered. I didn't know what the right answer was. I didn't want to scare her away.

I hope she calls me again. How can I explain what this is like? I think other people see it only as a "meet your mother or not" situation. They don't know what it means for my whole life. Today, though, I'm between worlds. Between never being someone and finally becoming someone.

But I'm isolated now. I feel bad that I'm shutting Bill out, even though he's the closest to me and the one I can tell everything to. But right now he seems so far away, in a different world. I think it is only temporary, but I don't know how to get him into my world, or if I even want him here.

December 4 After my birth mother called, I looked in the mirror and for the first time in my life I saw Japanese eyes that came from someone. From *her*. In the mirror I was seeing my mother for the first time. Now I know I came from somebody who exists; now I exist.

December 6 Today I walked to the store in the cold wind rain with no hat; I pushed my face into the wind and rain, and I felt powerful like when I was in Alaska. I saw my friend's face that I lost so long ago—he had smooth brown skin and long black hair—and I remembered how I used to look into his eyes and see myself. I'm neither white nor Asian, so I keep looking at people and wondering what it's like to be yourself. Now I'm really lost, and I can't find my birth mother anymore. I keep calling her on the phone but she doesn't answer.

December 16 It changes a lot of things in my life, just knowing she not only exists but is accessible. I'm so glad I found her. It's like a dam bursting. It's happy and sad and scary and joyful, and sometimes it's no big deal. It's everything and the opposite of everything.

January 7, 1992 Alyce's first Christmas. Why is that supposed to mean anything? Where was I on my first Christmas; where was my birth mother— was she thinking of me? Who was I with? Did I get any presents—where is my present—did I come with any possessions? Did she give me a toy, a blanket, a dress? Where is it? And who are all these people I spend Christmas with every year?

Who's my birth father? Did he cry? Does he get drunk on my birthday? Does he even know my birthday? Do I look like him? Is he funny? Does my child look like him? Who are his parents? Do we have the same mouth? Is he handsome?

Talked to my birth mother today, and we planned to meet in March. She said she wants to come up here, and she'll be calling me back. I did not enjoy talking to her today.

February 28 No word from her.

March 10 I've been putting off calling her, hoping she'll come through and call me, but doubting she will. Now I worry and wonder if she loves me. How can she not love me if she gave birth to me? How could she give me away if she loved me? As you can see, I'm in big trouble.

March 13 I called her yesterday. At first I thought we were going to have another awful and awkward telephone conversation, but then she said I was sweet for wanting to meet her, considering she had given me up for adoption and everything. She asked me if it bothered me that I was adopted. It was a great conversation. She even mentioned possibly telling her other children about me and said she would come up in April. She said she's getting more comfortable with me. So now I have to do more waiting. It had been two months since I last talked to her. Now I have to wait another month.

March 28 It's awful. I can't tell anyone. They know but are not thinking of it right now. I'm tired of saying *my* pain to everyone. People don't want to hear it. My pain is so confusing.

April 1 I've been so controlled all my life. People have made decisions for me, and now my birth mother is doing it again by not telling me who my father is; what right does she have to deny me my father? He's seventy-four years old and I've never known him, and she has the power to make sure I never do—he's *my* father after all.

Every few days or weeks I get really low, and it grows in my head and starts leaking out my eyeballs. I start pacing and making lists, and smiling at Bill when he talks to me so he'll think I'm listening to what he's saying.

April 20 I was trying to remember the last time I saw my mother. It was in December. It's hard to remember because I was only six days old. What was it like for her to hand me to the social worker? Did she cry? Did I cry? Did I look at her? Did she say anything to me? Did she give me anything? What was I wearing? She just handed me over like a piece of garbage. Here take this, I can't use it. She walked away and left me there. Who was holding me? Or was anybody holding me? Where did my mother go next? What did her body feel like? I was thinking maybe everybody was right, and I shouldn't have found her after all. I shouldn't have learned about what it really means to be adopted. She should have killed me then. I never would have felt all this. I can never forgive her completely. She can never love me enough. I will always hate her.

April 21 Called my birth mother today. She tried to put me off again, so Bill and Alyce and I are going down there to meet her. I was so shaky and scared. I hate this. I have to go through with it so I don't end up dead inside. Last night I hated her for giving me away. What will happen? How will she treat me? Am I doing the right thing? I am so scared. I've always thought I was tough; now I'm helpless and out of control.

How can Alyce grow up unscathed? Isn't every human being tortured by something? Will my love be enough for her? I touch her, hold her, kiss her, nurse her and play with her. But I can't get close enough. Will she feel loved? I do all that, yet she still turns away to go do something else, or still cries. Isn't a mother's love all anyone ever needs?

I want Alyce's love to make up for everything. I know that's a terrible burden to put on her. Her life is her own. It's to come. I am the past. But there's a place for us to be together. She won't reject me or give me up for adoption the way my mother did. I have to be sure of that.

If a child is abandoned by its mother, how can anything in life really matter?

April 24 Last night I dreamed I saw both my birth parents.

My birth mother was working in a little store in a mall. She was really pretty and young, in her forties or early fifties. She had big brown eyes and short, thick, slightly wavy black hair. Then I met my birth father. He was young, like my mother, and very handsome. He had brown eyes and wore glasses. We walked arm in arm, and I couldn't get over how handsome he was. I wanted desperately to see him and my birth mother together, to have a photo of them together and with me also. They went to a counselor together to try and work things out, not so they could be back with each other again but so they could get along and be in each other's lives. I was very happy. When I saw them, I thought they looked so good together, and I felt as if I belonged to them. I felt very lucky to have such beautiful parents.

April 26 All my life I forgot to look for my father.

April 29 If I can get through the next week of my life, I can get through anything. I'm going to meet my birth mother, and I can't believe it.

April 30 I feel sad to be leaving, like I'm going away and never coming back. I think things will never be the same. Part of me is dying. I'm afraid that when I come back I'll forget who I was before and just sit around trying to remember. I can't stop now, but I don't want to go. She will only hurt me. I've been packing and watching L.A. burn on the television because of the Rodney King verdict. It's all so perfect in a surreal sort of way.

May 5 Just back from one and a half hours with my birth mother. It was a perfect meeting!

We hugged.

I cried.

She said, "I knew this would happen," and gave me Kleenex.

I asked her to take her dark glasses off.
I stared at her.
She told me I was beautiful and perfect.

May 8 My visit with my birth mother was great. She was so kind, but I got only a taste of what it is to have a parent you're related to by blood. How grounding to look at who bore you and see yourself. It makes so much sense. How can people think it's unimportant? To have that every day of your life—what a treat it would be!

This woman who is my birth mother, but doesn't want to be, but can't help it, is small but very full and present. Her eyes look at you then look away. She looks very young.

I saw her trying to see me. I wanted to feel she was my mother, but I didn't feel it, I just knew it.

She is fighting her desires to get close to me. She doesn't want to tell me personal things—my birth father's name, my half sisters' and brother's names—but then she does. In some ways she was like a mother, and in some ways she was like a kid. I'm so glad she is normal and mature and not some bizarre or mysterious person.

I completely liked my birth mother, and I feel no malice toward her for giving me away. When we parted she looked at me and said, "I'm so sorry." I didn't know what to say. I didn't exactly know what she was sorry for.

I wonder if she'll call or write. I hope so; I'm afraid she won't though. I'm so glad I took Bill and Alyce with me, especially Alyce since it's her real grand-mother. Now Alyce has a line from both her parents and not just one.

May 9 I'm feeling more and more alone. It's okay—I think that's how it's supposed to be. Now I don't care as much about being alone. I miss Bill, but I can't control his life. He wants to get away from me every chance he gets. To go downstairs, to read a book, to watch TV. I'm sad that maybe we won't last. I'm tired. I wonder if he thinks we are coming apart, too. I'm so sad now that all I want to do is cry, but I'm so tired of crying. I was so high from meeting my mother, but now I just want to be a little baby and have someone take care of me. Everyone thinks I am so strong and brave and happy. They all want me to get on with my life, as if I can simply continue where I left off. But nothing's the same any more. I just want to go back to where I have real blood relatives and to where I was born. I want to go alone, but I have a child and I can't be away from her. Sometimes I wish I were free as I used to be.

When I look at my birth mother's picture, she looks so familiar. I have mixed feelings about her, loving her for being my mother and hating her for giving me away and for not accepting me fully into her life now. I feel cast away. No one can touch me.

My secret wish is to live in cars and motels my whole life.

Should I have done it? Does she want to see me again? Or will she bury me again? Oh, God.

June 29 I've been on hold, trying not to make any mistakes. Since I met her nothing in my life makes any sense. I'm trying to get better before any of this really matters. Not that I'm sick, but just different, and no one understands. Only Bill knows. Our families don't seem to understand, but our friends have been real supportive.

July 12 What I really want is for my mother to hold me in her arms. All I can do is hold Alyce. It's as close as I'm ever going to get.

July 22 Today I fantasized that I was walking down the street with my birth mother. What would that be like? Everyone would know she was my mother. I imagined it to be a wonderful experience, and at the same time I knew it would be untrue. Unfulfilling. Fleeting.

What is more pathetic than a motherless child?

September 9 I spoke to my real father two days ago. The fun just never ends. I called him but didn't identify my self as his daughter. Finally I mentioned my birth mother's name. There was an incredible pause while the world shifted on its axis, then he mumbled something about not knowing anything about it. I asked if I could call him back later, and he said yes. Then he hung up. I liked his voice though. I guess I'll write him a letter.

I'm sad, but at least I did it. I talked to my real father. I know by now it's just a dream and no matter what I get, none of it really matters. It doesn't matter if I know my birth parents or not, I still don't get them. It will never be real. It's too late. I got a million things I wanted, and I'm still not happy. Now I know I won't ever be happy.

It's only been two days since I called, but I've gone through the call enough in my head. It's very different from the way I felt about my birth mother. I don't know why I decided to call him, or how I got the guts. I think I almost didn't care any more, and just wanted to find him.

September 10 I'm walking around, and all these people are passing by, and they don't know that I've just talked to my real father for the first time in my life. They think I'm just shopping! I'm really somebody else, not who you think I am.

September 12   (I lost my father tonight)
Dear Sue,

I understand your concern, but I don't think that I can help you find the person you seek. If it is of interest to you, I myself am of Jewish descent. My father died of multiple sclerosis in his sixties; my mother died of arthritis in her eighties.

Your letter indicates that you are an intelligent and compassionate person. You write that you do not want to cause me trouble or disrupt my life. Unfortunately your phone call and letter have done just that. You are young and still have most of your life ahead of you. My wife and I are in our mid-seventies, married fifty-three years, and now our relationship is in a shambles because of this.

Please, no more calls or letters. I am trying to restore some semblance of harmony here for our remaining years, and more contact would certainly make things worse. Sincerely, J.M.

September 20   All of me is angry and all of me is relieved to have been in contact with my very own father.

November 20   I spent my whole childhood scrounging through my mother's drawers, cupboards and shelves. I was looking for anything with my name on it. She held the secrets to my life and told me I had no need of the information.

November 23   My thirty-fifth birthday is approaching. All it is to me is the one-year anniversary of my first contact with my birth mother.

She gave me to the social worker on Dec. 3. It's weird to think of myself as being passed from hand to hand, with each passing changing my entire life's history. I'm an imprisoned baby, wrapped up in a blanket so I can't break free, trapped so everyone can control me.

Living with Alyce is amazing. I've never lived with or even known a blood relative before. I can say for sure now that it is really different from living with nonrelatives. There's almost too much familiarity in the little nuances of her face and personality. This is a part of the human condition I had never experienced before. Ironically, it feels almost unnatural. And everyone knew about it except me. Life is not what I always assumed it was.

But it's the connection to my original family that ties me to the earth.

222

I want to know them and get a feel of my own self from them, but it's out of my reach. Someone told me it was too bad that all this had to happen right after I had a baby, because my depression kept me from enjoying my child. But I know that having Alyce was the only thing I could've done to begin the process I had denied for my whole life. Maybe that's why I put off having a baby for so long, because I knew it would do something like this to me. What I didn't know was how deeply it would do it.

December 8 Christmas is coming. I wish I knew if my birth mother was thinking about me. I wish she would talk to me. I want my brother and sisters.

I don't think God chooses certain children to be given to certain parents, just as I don't believe God chooses which shirt I buy off the rack. All children are perfect. Anyone could have been my parents. And anyone was.

February 5, 1993 I lost something that, until now, I never knew I had. I can't get it back and I can't relive any of the moments because I don't remember them and no one will tell me anything. I'm always running behind this death of my parents. I know they are dead, but then who are these ghost people alive and living other lives in Los Angeles? They just mock me and refuse to love me, while I can't help wanting to love them.

I want to hurry up and die so I can stop living this life and this lie. I want to scream, but I don't want anyone to hear me. I've been alone forever, hiding in my room. I'm trying to find an identity that's true, but it never works and I'm always a nothing and a nobody. How could you just throw me away? I was just a baby and look what you did to me. It's because of you I feel this way tonight. I had to pay for your shit.

June 23 I've been asking my adoptive mom questions about my childhood. The other night she told me I used to rock in my crib and bang my head so hard I would move the crib across the room. And she said I never slept more than thirty minutes at a time. At night I would repeatedly wake up and cry and she would have to rock me. That lasted until I was about three. It was hard to hear that about myself. I hate to picture that little screaming baby. And yet I keep asking for more and more because I want to know all of it.

June 29 I'm out here screaming to all my parents and relatives what I'm going through, and everyone just wants me to shut up.

July 17 Maybe I woke up every half hour so I wouldn't miss my mother when she finally came back for me.

August 26   Well, I'm pregnant again. I really wanted to have another baby, but now I have mixed feelings. I'm worried about what will happen this time. I've been waking up in the night and crying. I keep thinking about my childhood. I'm surprised I can function so well in the world, but it always feels like an act, or like something that will eventually go up in flames. Now my life has gone on for so long, I think maybe I will actually get through the whole thing.

November 9   I want to be totally honest with my children. I hated that my adoptive parents had secrets they wouldn't tell me. My adoption is like a big secret joke on me. I always pretended not to care so that no one would know how humiliating it was to be the butt of such a big joke.

November 28   Last night an hour before my birthday I woke up. Was she thinking of me? No. A thousand miles away I am dying while she sleeps. She doesn't even know my birthday. She blocked it out of her mind. How many people can say that?

November 29   Do we have to know our fathers to be happy?

December 1   I only want to be dead from Thanksgiving to New Year's. Is that so much to ask? She gave me away on December 3, when I was six days old. Where was I for two and a half months? My first Christmas is lost. No one will tell me where it is, but it's somewhere inside me, always mocking me. I know my first Christmas was not merry.

January 7, 1994   This pregnancy thing is really getting to me. I'm fine in the world, laughing and joking and living in some sort of denial, but having babies takes away my control, and I become at the mercy of others.

February 1   Alyce's third birthday. I'm worried about the upcoming birth. I've been working hard to make it a good birth. I'm scared of labor. I'm scared of having another Caesarean. But I have to be prepared just in case. I will not let this baby out of my sight. I feel more capable of giving birth now that I've met my own mother.

March 17   Eleven days since Jake's perfect birth. He was born right here at home. He came out of my body and right into my arms, and no one took him away.

Now my birth mother seems frozen in time. I wish I could know her better, but I have a more important future to look at. Alyce's birth forced me to search for her. I believe that finding and meeting my birth mother is what helped me feel human enough to give birth the normal and natural way. It was very important to me to have the baby and hold it for a long time. I know I wanted to make up for my own birth and relinquishment. In that way, Jake's birth was very healing.

December 10 My birth mother has kept me a secret from her new husband. Also from her three other children. She asked if I wanted to meet them, then she made excuses when I said, "Yes." When I finally found them, they sort of knew about me anyway. For a while my two half-sisters accepted me, but now they seem to have lost interest. My birth mother never tries to contact me. I went to my birth father's home, but he's no longer there. I met his ex-wife, and she was very kind, giving me pictures and telling me all about him. She said that my letter to her husband had made her realize that her whole married life was a lie. My letter gave her the energy, she said, to end her decades of unhappiness.

I know where my birth father is now, but I haven't tried to contact him again. She told their two sons about me and gave me their addresses. I wrote to them, and one wrote back a nice letter and sent pictures. That was the last I heard from him. After Jake's birth I sent each member of my original birth family a birth announcement. No one responded.

RUTH MYRA BAYER

Close By

I have four families. I grew up in a Jewish home, adopted by the parents I call my "real" parents, the ones who picked me up when I fell down, and sometimes still do. Three years after my "real" mom, Sarah, died, my father married a woman from the local Jewish community who had lost her husband. She and her four children became my second family.

Five years ago, my birth parents "found" me through the agency where I'd been adopted. We three met on a windy, bone-cold, rainy day in October. At the time, it seemed to me as if it were all happening to someone else, that I was just watching from close by. My birth mother, Annie, is American, distantly related to Emily Dickinson, so the story goes, and she grew up in New England. She has two children. My birth father, Michael, is Palestinian-American, also a native of New England, and he has five children. I was born to them when they were both twenty, with families who did not want them to be together.

In each of the families, I wanted to belong. My father and I knew ways of being with one another. These were not always smooth, but they were familiar. With everyone else it was new ground; they were not friends, and they were not family in the sense I knew it. The cultural conflict of my many families sharpened my vision, and I began to ask questions about my Judaism and about the conflict between Arabs, Palestinians, Israelis and Jews. I would never be able to return to my original comfortable acceptance of my unknown past, which is its own blessing and its own curse.

Many silences or cautions continue to exist in my new extended family. My adoptive parents don't acknowledge the existence of my birth parents. My birth parents are careful about telling the past, their short time together, my

225

coming-into-being. They were silenced long before, when I was conceived, because you did not talk about "that sort of thing" in 1958. I am careful, too, wary of hurting anyone with too much information or too many questions.

The fathers' stories are different from those of the mothers and are not easily blended. I call to mind two lands in which images of new and old knowledge attempt to find a balance. My adoptive father, who represents my adoptive family, is the old land, the one I have always known. My birth father is part of the new land. The lands are also Israel and Palestine. The mothers' stories are interwoven here. Their stories are about sorrow and loss and ways of loving.

Fathers

In the familiar land, the voices are the prayers I heard my grandfather murmur in the synagogue, while he swayed, facing east and inward. As he prayed, I braided the fringes of his prayer shawl. There is pride in the proverbs, stories and ancient heroines I know by name. I can recall the way my grandfather pinched my cheek or handed me a coin to put into the *tzedakah*, or charity box. The familiar is tender, with a steady eye on the importance of family, with a measured recognition of what is acceptable and good. This is an identity suffused with childhood memories, strengthened by the affection of my parents and by the receptive warmth of community. All of the words and events of the familiar are tangible, easily accessible.

In contrast, the new land is unknown, with voices that are not recognizable. Yet I see them as my ancestors. This land is new-born, dark, rough-edged, sometimes angry. Still it is a place to be cared for and to feel at home. This place is full of sisters and brothers, where my hands, my dark eyes, my gait and gestures are part of a pattern. There is passion, poetry and an old wildness. I cast about for an identity in this place. I learn the steps of the dance, but am not yet invited to join. I am drawn into the mystery of not knowing the name of the land or who will embrace me when I arrive.

One sunny morning, when I was in that early morning sleep where dreams are near the surface, I heard two voices in the room: one a Jew's, the other an Arab's. They were arguing the destiny of their people's, and I was in each of them and standing outside them as well, yearning to end the argument. I stretched my arms out to each of them in a pleading gesture, and without words, I asked them to stop their dispute. When I awoke I looked for them. The sunlight fell just where I'd imagined hearing the voices.

I dream sometimes of a place where Israel and Palestine, and my stories of family, do not reach me. I remembered my "real" father trying to sort out the story of my birth parents, wanting all at once not to lose me, but to be accepting of my discovery. He'd grown up the first generation American-born, learning Yiddish as his first language, hearing stories of the "old country" all through his youth. When I told him of my birth father's background, he found a way to connect his own life with that of Michael's, saying, "Oh, he's the son of immigrants as well." It's just a coincidence, but for a short time my adoptive grandfather and my birth grandfather lived in the same town in New England, both trying to find their place in America as newcomers.

The New Land: My Birth Father

My birth father had phoned his youngest son late one night after a violent spring storm six years ago. He explained that he'd had a daughter twenty-nine years earlier. He said he'd been standing in the window of his home in the mountains and seen lightning strike close by, and had known it was time to tell his children of my existence, time to find me.

Ten years later, my birth father, Michael, and his youngest son, Alex, asked me to meet them at the airport before their flight to Israel/Palestine. We'd come to know one another through infrequent visits and occasional phone calls. Whenever I spoke with Michael I could be direct, unlike with my dad, but I was uneasy still. I felt I had taken steps to get to know him, but he had stayed in the same place, letting me do the work. I didn't know at that moment that I'd be stepping into a new land . . . onto a field of stones and generations-old olive trees.

Alex was nineteen, the age his father had been when I'd been conceived. He was so optimistic and bright-eyed, waiting in the airport, wearing his black leather bomber jacket, his loafers and his black leather knapsack like his father's. The Father, as he liked to call himself, smoked and drank coffee in the way of his cousins across the sea, impatient to depart, full of idealism for a reunion. I can never mother or sister them, I realized as we three stood talking. I am always separated, sometimes by politics, sometimes by Michael's distant manner. Yet this is the father who'd pushed for contact, talking my birth mother into writing a letter to the adoption agency so that they could in turn legally contact me.

A month later I called Michael to welcome him home, excited to hear news of his—my—Palestinian family. Michael spoke small talk at first. "How are you?" "What's new?"

I answered, sensing some awkwardness I couldn't yet identify, and then asked, "Michael . . . so . . . how was Israel . . . or Palestine?"

"Do you really want to know?"

I didn't see the significance of this remark and instead leapt into the fire, heart first. "Yes, of course, I . . ."

"Fine, fine. Do you want to hear about the children held in detention without trial for months? Do you want to know about how the soldiers bull-doze houses and arrest husbands and sons? Do you want to hear about the rubber bullets and the tear gas, or maybe you want to know about all of the olive groves that were destroyed?"

I couldn't back out of this, and I didn't know where I was going either. This land was angry, trembling with a pain I did not yet understand. At night I dreamed about the two lands, touched the fertile soil of each one with my hands, walked between their trees, navigated a careful path to the houses of both of my fathers.

"The Jews here are apathetic. Even my colleagues, they just stop talking to me when I bring up the conflict. What does your dad do; nothing but give more money to the Israelis. You, too, you don't know anything. What did you read? The real history isn't in the books you read."

With the sound of his voice there was the scent of carob in my room. I could see a field of newly planted olive saplings. The summer air became cool. There was the sound of bleating goats and the crying of a small child. The images were of the new and the old land, borrowed from all I'd learned. In the distance I could hear the tiring pace of heavy boots and the click of the catch being released on the trigger of a gun. I simply wanted to sit with my birth father, to look at photographs of our ancestors, to hear stories of his parents and grandparents.

"You're just like everyone else. Like all the Jews in this country. You pre-tend there is no Palestinian people. You can't be any kind of Palestinian; you're a Jew."

The sound was muffled, like the woods after a snowfall. I felt alone. I wanted to hear some sound to welcome all of who I am. I heard no marching, no trains, no children crying. I strained to listen for a reassuring footfall, a step in the dance, a note of some old song. I answered.

"Michael . . . I . . . can we? . . . maybe when you aren't so angry, we can . . ."

The phone was slammed down. It would be months before we would be in touch again, and I would feel an urge to keep Michael at arm's length for a long time. My heart hung there, the light of day collected on the wood floor. The field of fragile saplings disappeared as well. In its place was a stone temple, with walls of mosaics, and at the entrance, a dusty old man.

The Old Land: My Father

Five years after I'd met my birth parents and discovered my cultural origins,

I decided it was time to travel to Israel and Palestine. When I first told my parents about the trip, they didn't appear to be upset, but two weeks later when I was at my parents' home for a family event, my dad, with a very uncharacteristic stiffness, asked me to come into his study. I moved papers and mail to make room for myself on the couch and sat down. My dad then declared that he did not want me to go on this trip. "It's dangerous, you don't know the people, you're going to dangerous places, and I'd really rather you didn't go."

I reassured him that I did know one of the co-leaders of the tour through very trustworthy old friends and that some of the members of the trip were even his age. "Dad, maybe it's more dangerous than going to Europe on a tour, but this is something I need to do. I've waited a long time to go back to Israel because I began to feel that what the Israelis were doing was wrong. I promised myself that I would go only if I could talk to both Palestinians and Israelis."

"I don't understand. You used to believe in Israel. You know what happens there. People get killed every day, especially tourists. You can't go wondering off somewhere." This was the same father who had slept with one eye open when I went out with friends in high school, who'd ask me twenty questions before I went away on a trip and who'd stayed by my side in the hospital when I was twenty-eight years old. "I don't know why you're doing this."

He wasn't talking just about protecting his daughter or making sure I'd call him once a week while I was away. He was deeply afraid for me, and he could not understand why I would take, what were to him, serious risks.

"Dad, I'm going because I have to see with my own eyes. It is because you taught me about human dignity and the preciousness of life. These are your values."

He could not reply. I'd realized long ago that those "values" had a limited application. Arabs were excluded. I made no exclusions.

My father had escaped many times through silence. This time he'd chosen to speak up. I knew it had not been easy for him. This was the same father who could not say aloud that my mom had committed suicide although everyone else knew. He had not been able to face the seriousness of her illness because he had loved her too much. Sometimes he would feign forgetfulness about memories of my childhood because they reminded him of my mother. His brother had been killed serving as a doctor in World War II and he had watched his mother refuse to take her insulin following the death of this eldest son. She, too, had died. I could understand how much he had hurt in his life and how much loss he had suffered. Still, I was not able to understand how a loving father could not trust that his own daughter was telling truths.

But then, we are often only able to see the truths we want to see.

When I returned from my trip my father asked questions. I didn't know if he was just being polite or was genuinely curious, so I prefaced my answers with, "Are you sure you really want to know?" I told him about the refugee camps, about the suppression of political organizing and the closing of schools, about the poverty and the forced unemployment in the Occupied Territories.

He answered, "The Arabs (it was as if he could not pronounce the word 'Palestinian') are uneducated, so they stay where they are. How can you expect them to find work if they are uneducated? And then those who have gone to other Arab countries to work forget they ever had families. These people aren't taking care of their own. They'll stay in those camps if they don't try to help themselves."

I was silenced once again by the appalling prejudice. I knew my father to be a generous, kindhearted man, very involved in his religious and city communities, and I had hoped that he would trust what I'd seen, that he'd see beyond his own racism. I recalled my stepmother's constant refrain: "You didn't live here during the Holocaust; you don't know what Israel means to Jews who survived. The Arabs want to throw us into the sea."

I didn't tell my father about meeting my cousins, my Palestinian cousins. I didn't tell him that I looked like my youngest cousin, with her dark hair and eyes and her smile. I kept silent about their kindness, about how my elder cousin had been jailed for three years, without trial, for political meetings held in his home or how his wife needlepointed all of the upholstery in her living room as a way of safeguarding her own peace of mind while her husband was imprisoned. I saw their garden, with its roses and pepper plants, chickens and vegetables, created during the *Intifada*, or uprising, so as to develop independence from the occupation. I understood more about the human family, and my own longing to belong, in that one hour with my cousins than I had in my entire lifetime. My elder cousin told me, "When you return to Palestine, you will be welcome in our home."

Mothers

In the fall we nearly lost Annie. I was not ready to lose another mother. Even the word had become precious to me, as if savoring its letters and the sound would keep my mothers alive. All that time visiting my birth mother, Annie, in the hospital, riding back and forth, forty-five minutes each way, I'd been trying to place her among the many characters and events in my life. When I faced Annie, I also faced my mother, Sarah, and her death. I wanted to give Annie a location, a room in my mind where she and I both would be comfortable.

Annie had been found curled up in a ball with what was discovered to be a brain aneurysm. My half-sister, Annie's daughter, Karen, talked of how, fifty or a hundred years ago, Annie would most certainly have died; this would have been her time. I, who usually prefer to honor the natural world, was relieved that we have taken to searching minds with video cameras and finding the "demons" inside. My "real" mother, Sarah, had lived with illness and pain for twelve years before finally taking her own life, a mother's second leaving for me. Annie's illness had come without warning and could have quickly taken her, leaving me, for the third time, without a mother.

The waiting time while Annie was in surgery was the most difficult. I suddenly remembered details of the aftermath of my mother's suicide. My father had phoned me in France, where I was studying for a year. He was advised to tell me she was suffering from a coma so that I would come home to be with her, yet still be able to contemplate the possibility that she would die before I arrived. During the flight I recognized the possibility of her imminent death. I rode from the airport, two and a half hours away from my home, with family friends, who could not speak for fear of betraying my father's wishes to tell me himself. In front of the house were several cars, there for the impending funeral. Later I would recognize all the signs, but I was newly born into this particularly cruel realm of loss and could not see what was so obvious.

No one ever actually declared that her death had been a suicide, and my father adamantly denied it. But all the hints were there, and friends of the family quietly told me of her terrible pain and of her honesty about the toll it had taken on her and on her family. It was many years before I was actually able to unravel truths about my mom's leave-taking.

When Annie was in the hospital I wanted to know everything about her illness, her surgery, her recovery. I hungered for details to make up for those I was never allowed to know about my mom's sickness and death. I wanted to know how Annie's surgery was done, how they cut and entered the brain, how they found the clot, what the future held, how the genetics of all this fit into my own life. Karen was my spy and my connection. Sweetly, though with fear herself, she would phone me on the days I couldn't come to visit, and when I did visit, she would be with me at Annie's bedside.

A week after surgery Annie requested that we take photos of her. She still had staples holding her scalp together, and her hair was growing back in patches of blonde. She looked all at once beautiful and sad. When she'd first come out of surgery, her face had been taut and her eyes appeared sunken and so green. The starkness of her features shocked me—I was reminded of photos of Holocaust survivors, their bodies emaciated, their faces holding onto whatever small spark of life remained.

She wanted us to be sure to photograph the staples, and as we pulled flowers from the vases on the windowsill and put them behind her ear, we all giggled. Annie put one of the flowers in her mouth like a flamenco dancer. Still, she looked weak, her face pale and bewildered from all of the medications and after effects of the surgery.

Karen and I took turns posing for the pictures with Annie. The week before I'd bought a book on Mary Cassatt for Annie, and the photos we took that day resembled Cassatt's paintings—physical closeness and poignant tenderness between mother and daughter. We called our photos "the Mary Cassatt after-surgery masterpieces."

This was not the mother of my knee-skinning days, who worried when I was riding "no-handed" on my bike, knew when I was telling ferocious lies and hugged me proudly for every "A" I received in school. I had not been ready to lose again, as Annie had left me once in my infancy, and as I'd lost my adopted mother to her pain in my young womanhood. Now here Annie was, helpless for the moment, unable to be the support that she'd been since I'd met her—like my mother, whose illness had not permitted her to be a complete mother for many years. I knew I still wanted some of that mother-likeness from Annie, though to my friends I denounced her as my mother, telling myself and them that I was now independent and that I'd had my "real" mother; I didn't need another one.

Usually I visited Annie with Karen nearby. Sometimes we would take turns staying in the room, both of us wanting time alone with her, but pleased to spend time with one another as well. I went to the hospital only once when I knew Karen wouldn't be there. Karen had given her mother a pair of lovely earrings, and Annie wanted to put them on. I handed her the box.

"I hope I can get them in the holes. I usually use a mirror."

She managed to put the left earring in with only a little hesitation, but the second one wouldn't go in.

"Here, you do it, Ruth. I can't get it in."

I hesitated. This was the side of her head where the surgery had been done. I was still squeamish about the sight and the antiseptic smell, and I'd had limited physical contact with Annie. We hugged, but it was Karen who massaged her back, rubbed her feet, and was comfortable touching Annie's scalp where her skull had been opened.

I took the earring and tried to get it in the tiny hole.

"I can't. You'll do it better than I will. I don't want to poke you with it."

"Try it again. I can't do it. You'll have to. Anyway, you ought to get used to it."

Her tone was sharp. I froze momentarily. The earring went in on the third or fourth try but I was stunned. Get used to what, I thought? A mother who is in pain? Taking care of someone I love? Helping someone who is incapacitated? She did not know me at all. Stepping back, I understood that Annie was homesick, bedsore, exhausted and tense. She had wanted to go home, but she'd just been told she'd have to stay a few more days for observation. I knew she spoke from terrible discomfort, but I too wanted to go home, or to have home come to me.

Feeling myself about to cry, I gave her a hug, gathered up my winter coat and said a gracious good-bye. The ride home was tearful, angry. Thirty-some years of *"where were you when I was a child and growing up?"* and *"don't you know I already had one sick mother?"* and *"who are you to tell me what to get used to?"* were given voice in that journey. I recognized these messages as old friends and, though for Annie's part, there was no such complex meaning intended, her words caught me, lodged between my two mothers.

My mothers were women who lived their lives and their decisions with inner strength. Sarah chose a sunny day to decide her way, after years of no control over her body. She went out to the little camp we owned by the lake and rested in the sun. I have often wondered what she would have thought of Annie, or Michael and me together after all these years. Annie, the one who had shared her body with me, had to continue her young life and was given the only acceptable option at the time. She tells of the six months apart from her family, pregnant, among other women in her situation who were making the best of terrible circumstances. Her father told her to forget the birth had ever happened. She moved forward, though never quite leaving it behind. In the first year of our meeting, Annie wrote a letter to my father. She did not send it. She told him that he'd been a good parent, that she wished she could have given me more and that she hoped that one day they would meet.

There is still uncertainty between Annie and me. I come and go with her, perhaps more content to make the decision to take leave myself than to have it made for me as it was in the past.

With Annie as with most everyone in my families there is some moment of leaving; I must leave some part of myself behind and choose to speak only as a Jew, only as a Palestinian, only as a child by birth or only as a child by adoption. I am, however, all of these wrapped into one. I do not want to give any of them away.

One Land

What is the name of this land? It has no borders, no lines stopping people from exchanging news, trading, marrying, telling stories. It appears too simple, too impossible. The people struggle with birth and death still, with anger and love, but they do not build fences, they do not covet the other's trees, women, or ground. I hear the footsteps of ancestors approaching; old, dignified women, and stubborn, hardworking men, with no secrets.

LAURA CUNNINGHAM

Sleeping Arrangements

There are still missing pieces. The family history must forever remain incomplete. Had my mother lived, I feel she would have told me about my father. Because I was eight years old when she died, I was left with the version she chose to tell a child: the saga of the handsome hero, lost in a war.

Who was Larry? What really happened? When I asked my uncles for more information, they could not even verify the spelling of his last name. "We just don't know." Hadn't they asked Rosie? No, they said, they had not. They respected her privacy. If nothing else, we are a discreet family.

My mother was thirty-five years old when I was born. She made her own way, she made her own choice. It was only the time and tradition that forced her to create a fiction.

My question today is: Why did she create so elaborate a fiction? When I imagine Larry fighting a war, with a dog at his side, I have to laugh. Rosie, why did you include a boxer (not even a German shepherd) in this strange legend?

Growing up, I exchanged one fantasy for another: My father was alive somewhere. I could find him. I added to my mother's story and created a dozen alternative endings:

I was always walking into my father's office (still the sun-bleached war office) and surprising him. Having seen too many B movies, I ran with what clues I had.

In my mind, the melodramas unfold: I arrive by train in a strange southern town, to kick up dust. Why do I wear all white and that slouch hat? To me "the South" meant *Gone with the Wind* or *A Streetcar Named Desire*.

235

I proceed—from the dusty street—to his office, or, better yet, an antebellum porch, where my father and I can fling ourselves into delicate frenzies of regret.

What actually happened was not romantic or melodramatic—it was tedious. I wrote to the Hall of Records. My letter was returned, stamped INSUFFICIENT INFORMATION. I wrote again: How many Larry Moores could have been stationed in Miami in 1946? Too many, I was told. I would need the missing man's consent before his file could be released. Later requests to every imaginable authority were also denied. My father's name was too common. I would have to give up.

I almost did. My efforts became erratic. I might not think of him for months, then I would see an out-of-state phone book and flip to his name. That was how I conducted my search—standing up, in fluorescent telephone "communications centers." Uncertain even of the spelling, I worked the combinations: Moore, Lawrence; More, Laurence; even Mawr, Laurenz. I studied the listings: Larry Moore of Flat Creek Road?

Mentally, I traveled to Flat Creek Road and there he was—Larry Moore, standing on his porch. He stares, brooding over a bourbon and the muddied waters of Flat Creek. In this scenario, his wife walks onto the veranda holding an empty vase. "Why, who's that, Larry?" she asks.

"No one," he answers, his eyes meeting mine.

My only problem with this version is that I rebel at its maudlin nature. I don't like melodrama. It might be my life, but it's not my material.

I never had the nerve (or perhaps the need) to telephone any of the hundreds of Laurence/Larry/Lawrence Moore/More/Mawrs. The closest I came was to draft a letter to be copied. "Dear Laurence/Larry/Lawrence, Were you perhaps stationed in Miami in 1946?" I explained that this was not "an emotional matter" but simple curiosity on my part. There would be no unpleasant scenes. It was not a case of anguish, I wrote, then realized I had misspelled the word "anquish."

Squish.

I never finished the letter, never copied it, never mailed it. Still, the potential drama lurks never too distant at the back of my mind.

Hope is sneaky; it hides behind reason. As recently as three years ago I might pause at a communications center to flip under the M's in the book marked "Alabama."

Then I stopped. Just quit. I don't want to do it anymore. I ask my Uncle Len to "tell me the story of how he looked" one last time.

Uncle Len and I sit in the garden of his cottage in Florida, a tropical place, redolent of gardenias and citrus, a place not so far from where Len actually saw Larry. Uncle Len tells the tale, as best he can recall it.

"I had gone with Rosie to the ballroom of the old Grenada Hotel. It was very crowded inside. I can still see the dance floor, so packed with people they couldn't really dance—they just moved in place. And Rosie became very excited. She stood up on tiptoe and said, 'There he is, there he is . . . That's him.' I looked across the crowd—and it seemed to me that she was pointing out a blond man, but he was facing the other way. I saw his hair; it was very fair . . . sort of sandy. He was nicely dressed and seemed to be a good dancer. But, before I could get a closer look, he disappeared into the crowd—not *deliberately* leaving, just being caught up in that great crush of bodies on the dance floor—and then he was gone."

Even this "documented" glimpse of Larry is characteristically fleeting. I swear to myself never to ask Uncle Len to repeat this story. His dark eyes, so like my mother's, shine with unshed tears. His voice is softer even than usual, halting. "Oh," he added, "I do remember . . . one more . . . detail. He was wearing a sweater, a special kind of sweater that was in style then . . . and Rosie told me he liked that style."

Uncle Len takes an important pause—he's delivering the goods. The final fact gleaned about my father: "He wore cardigans."

Now *that* . . . is my material. I say good-bye to fair-haired Larry in his cardigan and swear not even to think of him, but to use the time and energy on someone else. These days, I limit my Larry thoughts to filling in the blanks on "biography" questionnaires. Where it says "Father's Name," I write "Laurence Moore" (most likely spelling), and after "Father's Occupation," I scribble "Aviator." (Why lose the entire legend?)

His absence may have benefitted me more than his presence. If my early life's a fiction, well then, fiction is my trade.

The truth, I feel, is something stronger. I was raised by two men who cared for me, and raised me, against convention. I'm their child, not his. And I owe my existence not to him but to my mother, who risked more than usual to give me life. It was my mother's love that made me. I am my mother's daughter. I am hers.

What I may have missed by not having the usual set of parents I can never know. Certainly I gained great love and benefitted from being raised not merely by men but by those two special men. As a bonus, I may have been given an appreciation of the uniqueness inherent in all human connections. What else I may have gained—or escaped—I'm still discovering.

PATRICIA FOX

Journey into the Past

I had always known my birth father was Scottish, with red hair and blue eyes, and that my birth mother was French, a brunette with blue eyes. My adoptive parents had not been told much, but they had always shared all these little bits of information with me. The only medical knowledge we had was that my maternal grandmother was diabetic.

I had contacted The Good Samaritan Agency in Lewiston, Maine, the previous year and the agency had sent me some additional "non-identifying" information. I now knew that I had been born at 9:55 P.M. and that my mother was single, had dropped out of school as a high-school freshman and was the youngest of nine children; my father had graduated from high school, was then working as a "coating machine operator" and was married. I also learned from these records that my maternal grandmother was a Native American who had never attended school and was fifty-seven years old at the time of my birth. Her husband, then sixty-seven, was a woodsman.

Like a novelist constructing the perfect plot, I had coincidentally found my birth mother, Raymonde, only a month before, on Mother's Day. The search for my mother, like my own gestation, had taken nine months. After sending her a letter introducing myself—signing my birth name, Kathleen, at the suggestion of my adoption search support group—she had called me immediately.

My husband, Rick, answered the phone that evening in May. He handed it to me with a look of surprise. "Patty, it's *her* (she had asked for Kathleen). She has a soft, sweet-sounding voice," he whispered in my ear, smiling reassuringly. Although French is Raymonde's native language, she has a strong command of English, so we had no difficulty communicating.

Without a moment of hesitation she told me how she had first met my birth father in Madawaska, Maine, when she was seventeen years old and he was thirty-two. She said my father had been divorced, living with his mother and his nine-year-old son and not interested in another marriage. When she became pregnant with me two years later, my father drove her to a foster home in Bangor two hundred miles away, where she lived until I was born.

She said that my father had visited her only once while she was in the home and then severed their relationship. Devastated, my teenage mother, after a long deliberation, gave me up for adoption and went home to Canada. Her choice of words and the tone of her voice conveyed a lingering bitterness with this old boyfriend, and when we met in Montreal a few weeks later, she was openly disappointed: "You look like your father," she said, as she flashed me a strained smile. While there, I also met her three children, all in their twenties: two women, each single with one child, and a divorced man with two daughters. One of my half-sisters whispered to me, "It was good that you were brought up by someone else."

I found myself initiating all of the questions. She did not appear interested in the woman I had become. Nor was she interested in my children, her own grandchildren. Nevertheless, everyone was excited and welcoming. Still I left our reunion with a feeling of emptiness, longing for the "instant connections" I had read about in other people's stories.

A few weeks later, Raymonde, drunk and crying, called me in the early hours of the morning. "You have a sister, Lizette, who was born two years before you. She is your father's child, too. Find her!" For almost an hour she alternated between tears and venomous remarks about my father. During a later call, she admitted she had given up this first child to her own sister. "Don't tell her, because my sister told me not to cause any more trouble." Today my aunt's phone number is still in my desk drawer: I haven't known what to do with this information. What if my aunt has never told Lizette that she was adopted? Do I have the right, the need or the obligation to bring this bit of news into Lizette's life?

I also put my father's phone number in my desk drawer, letting it sit there as my possession before trying to make any contact with him. Once Raymonde had given me his name, Clifford MacWhinnie, and told me that he probably still lived in the town where they had dated thirty-four years before, all I had to do was find his name in the phone book. Knowing that he had never seen me before, and fearing he might deny his paternity, I carefully constructed a short but succinct letter explaining my existence.

"Dear Mr. MacWhinnie: This might come as quite a shock to you, but I am your daughter." My letter went on to explain that I was a high school

English and Theater instructor and married with two children. I indicated that my family was planning a camping trip up north, near his home, at the end of June and asked if we could meet. I enclosed a wallet photo of myself to help erase any doubts he might have about our genetic connection. A week passed without a response, but I held my impatience in check until Father's Day. It was early evening when I locked myself in my bedroom, having told no one of my intention, and dialed the number. What a disappointment when I reached an answering machine. Later, I tried again. "Hello," a raspy voice answered.

"Hello, Mr MacWhinnie. This is Pat Fox. Did you receive my letter?" I said, the beat of my heart pounding in my ear.

A slight pause . . . then, "Yes, I did."

I breathed a sigh of relief. I wasn't in the mood to break the news of my existence over the phone. Another awkward pause while I waited. The paradoxical nature of the situation left me tongue-tied. This stranger was my father. I needed to choose my next words carefully. I wanted to know everything. I wanted him to like me, to be proud of me. I needed to know about his life and if we had any similarities. Yet he could hang up on me at any moment. He might even deny his responsibility in my creation. Happily, however, he continued speaking, directing the course of our conversation.

"Your letter gave me a variety of emotions: happiness, sorrow, anger. I was quite shocked. I have many questions I would like to ask you, but the phone isn't the way to do it."

I experienced another wave of relief: he was not going to reject me or his connection to me. Afraid to lose momentum, I took the plunge. "Will it be possible for my family and me to come up and meet you when I mentioned?" I held my breath, feeling my stomach twitter with anxiety.

"I just wrote you a letter. I'm sorry to disappoint you; I'm afraid that won't be possible. I'm having company at that time."

"Oh . . ." was all I could squeeze out. Was he lying? I wondered.

Sensing my disappointment, and perhaps eager to change the subject, he asked, "Tell me, how is your health?"

Touched by a sincerity and concern I had not encountered with my birth mother, I responded with candor and found myself describing my recent problems with allergies.

"Well, let me tell you where that all comes from," he explained.

I grinned inwardly, realizing I had scored. It was his way of indicating I was his. He proceeded to expound on the numerous medical adversities he had encountered over the years, from high blood pressure and glaucoma to allergies and other breathing difficulties. To him they were a list of bothersome problems, but to me they signaled that for the first time in my life I would be able to fill out my own family medical history form. I began to forgive him for not allowing us to meet. Somehow the conversation soon took a turn to our driving skills, and I admitted my tendency to have a lead foot.

"You have someone to take after there, as I have been known to go a little fast myself," he chuckled. I thought I could detect a hint of pride in his voice.

I remember thinking that I liked this man, my father, and I felt a connection. With renewed confidence, I approached another important subject.

"You have a son, Tommy." It was more of a statement than a question. "Is he the only child you have?"

When he said yes, I was glad in a very selfish way. This meant I was now the only daughter he was in contact with, and I felt the possibilities of a relationship between us increase.

Memories of our remaining conversation are hazy, but I recall spurts of spontaneous laughter from both of us, while I lounged on my bed like a teenager. As our conversation was drawing to a close, I bravely asked when we could meet. "When my company leaves," he said. It sounded hopeful. Still, I hung up without wishing him a happy Father's Day; I wasn't bold enough for that.

I tried not to obsess too much about this unfolding drama, but that didn't stop me from sharing it with interested friends. On Tuesday his letter arrived. There were several things about it that made an impression on me: His handwriting was unexpectedly embellished for a male, and his vocabulary indicated a level of education I had not expected.

To say that I was greatly surprised would be putting it mildly. . . . Naturally I am anxious to meet you. . . . I'm at a loss for words at the moment as I have so many questions to discuss. . . . I'll have to get in touch with you later this summer and set up a meeting that will be compatible for all. I realize you may be disenchanted by this tentative schedule, but I have no choice.

His letter increased my desire to meet him and allayed any reservations I had concerning his intentions. However, on the back side of the stationery, almost as an afterthought, his tone switched from polite to scolding: "Did you consider that your letter could have fallen into someone's hands who might have been very hurt and unforgiving? There is no need for more hurt . . . especially at this stage and time in life. Do you agree?" This addendum left me confused and defensive. I was determined to address it in our next conversation. My chance came sooner than expected. At noon on Friday of the same week, the phone rang. I recognized the voice immediately, a deep hoarse tone with that slight trace of a French accent, common to people of northern Maine.

I don't remember what excuse he gave for calling, but I remember blurting, "Has your company left yet?"

"No . . ." he answered with a slight chuckle at the forwardness of my question. Anxious to exonerate myself of the accusations in his recent letter, I asked, "Since you seemed upset about the contents of my letter getting into the wrong hands, would you have preferred a phone call?"

"No," he answered.

"Well, how about a knock at your door?" Naturally his answer was the same.

Apparently he appreciated my decision once I had pointed out my other options, because our conversation quickly proceeded with ease. He told me that his ninety-three-year-old mother was dying in a nearby nursing home. He also told me about his Boston terrier, Pepper. As he shared a few stories, it was obvious that his attachment for his dog was deep. Our affinity for dogs is mutual, and I described to him our golden retriever, Annie. Then, I asked him if he had remained a coating machine operator at the paper mill.

He laughed at my innocence. "I became the superintendent of a large section of the Fraser Paper Mill, but I'm retired now and have been for quite some time." He spoke at length about his various promotions, and I listened just for the simple pleasure of being able to hear my father's voice. I was proud to be connected to such a successful man and was grateful for the gift of this call, but disappointed that our meeting had been postponed again.

I waited almost two more weeks before I called him a second time. I was determined to set a date for our meeting. He admitted that his company had left, but was hesitant about letting me and my family come to meet him. Every idea I had was met with a negative response. It was not possible to meet at his home because he did not want anyone else to see us. I knew he lived alone because my search had taken me to the town historian, who was able to fill me in on his present status. "I thought you lived alone," I accused. He was surprised at my knowledge, but added vaguely that there were other people involved who might appear. He was adamant about not being discovered. I assumed his need for secrecy meant that he was filled with guilt and shame.

Still I remained relentless in offering ideas that would meet his need for privacy. His attempts to discourage me finally failed, or perhaps he let me find a solution because a part of him also wanted this meeting. In any event, it was done. He agreed to meet me and my family in just four days at a campground outside his hometown.

As we set off to drive the four hundred miles to the northernmost tip of

Maine, I smirked, realizing that this was the one area of Maine I had always said I would never visit. Anything north of Bangor seemed barbaric and desolate.

The morning of our meeting I awoke early with a nervous knot of fearful anticipation in my stomach. We drove the last thirty miles of the journey and arrived at the campground just a half hour away from my father's home. After settling in, I entered the campground office to make my call. I was so excited, my throat was dry and I could barely speak.

"Hello, Mr. MacWhinnie. This is Pat. I am here at the campground."

Before I could say anything else, he asked for the location of our campsite, responded to my directions with a curt "OK" and hung up. He hadn't told me if or when he would arrive. Back at the campsite, I sat and waited. Chewing what few nails I had left, I anxiously watched each approaching car. I was worried I would encounter another failed connection.

It wasn't long before I noticed a beige car slow down and pull in bearing a solitary driver wearing a white golf cap. I strained to catch a glimpse, but the reflection of the sun off the window prevented me from seeing more. I was alone. Rick had taken the children to the waterfront, allowing me some privacy for this moment. With a slight hesitation, I stood up from my chair, uncertain of what to say, feeling every beat of my heart resounding from my throat to the pit of my stomach. He rolled the window down and asked, "Do I have the right place?"

I replied, "I think so."

He emerged from the car, and words were not necessary as we embraced and both let out a sob. He broke away and looked up at me. "My, you're a fine-looking woman."

I blushed, uncomfortable but pleased with the compliment. I must have thanked him, but I don't recall much of the specifics of the conversation, only bits and pieces. My children appeared bearing grins, not fully comprehending the undercurrent of emotions. He embraced them also and shook Rick's hand. Then he guided my nine-year-old son, Cory, and my six-year-old daughter, Alyson, onto his lap like a long-lost friend and won them over with smiles and contagious enthusiasm. My husband stayed in the background with his quiet but strong support. Soon everyone's cameras appeared, and we all started taking pictures. I asked him to take off his sunglasses so that my suspicion about our strong resemblance could be confirmed. When he replied by whipping them off, I encountered twinkling blue eyes that mirrored my own.

"I think I look like you," I said hesitantly. He didn't deny it and willingly posed with me for the next picture. After a short while, Rick took the kids away again to allow me more time with this stranger, my father.

Soon he took a photo album out of the car and proudly showed me pictures of his prized woodworking projects—end tables, chalet clocks and decorative shelves—along with his culinary masterpieces of elaborately decorated cakes.

Later he asked me how I had found Raymonde and then his address. In detail, I began to describe my nine-month search that had uncovered my biological roots.

My first success took place when my adoptive mother and I were granted permission to look at my original birth certificate in the probate court in Lewiston. For the first time, I saw my birth mother's name, although she had signed the certificate Ramona Berube rather than Raymonde. From there I traced my own hospital records, in which I uncovered an old address for one of my birth parents in Madawaska. An Aroostook County phone book, covering the greater part of sparsely populated northern Maine, included over sixty listings for "Berube." Every night for three weeks, I would pick up the phone and begin calling complete strangers, hoping to discover one of my birth mother's nine brothers or sisters.

My line was always the same: I was doing genealogical research. I found many helpful people, including one man who referred me to a Berube Family genealogy expert in Connecticut, who then gave me the numbers of two other family genealogists in Canada.

On the assumption that my birth mother might be a French-Canadian who had been living in Maine when she met my father, I had also written to the U.S. Bureau of Immigration and Naturalization to see if she had ever applied for working papers in the United States. When that turned out to be a dead-end, I refiled an information request with the INS asking for information about my maternal grandmother, Victoria, who had co-signed my mother's medical forms at the time of my delivery in Bangor. The INS was able to give me the name of my maternal grandfather, who had once entered the United States on a work visa as a woodsman, along with two daughters, Raymonde and a second whose name was mysteriously crossed out.

One of the Canadian Berube genealogy researchers was then able to find the family line in his records. Pretending that I was hosting a mammoth family reunion, I asked for a list of telephone numbers of living descendents, including my birth mother's, and then got her address by calling the Montreal operator. Counting phone calls, administrative filing fees and travel, my search cost me about five hundred dollars and five hundred hours of my life.

After hearing my detective story, "Mac" invited us all to lunch in Caribou, a town thirty miles southeast of the campground. I suspected this long-distanced lunch spot was to avoid any chance encounters with people he might know. We drove off in his car, with me in the front passenger seat and my family and Annie in the back.

"Have you thought much about me over the years?" I asked bravely as he maneuvered the car along the curving road through rough virgin wilderness.

After a pause, he answered me with a choked voice and eyes shiny with tears: "I thought it had been all taken care of."

A slap in the face couldn't have stunned me more. I was to have been aborted. Although this did not match Raymonde's version of my birth story, I decided not to question this discrepancy for now. Also I had detected regret and shame in his voice, so at least I knew that he cared. After a few miles of awkward silence, I began chatting, trying to indicate some kind of forgiveness for his past actions or his initial hesitancy toward me.

"Your mouth moves just like Tommy's!" he shouted, almost going off the road. He also remarked on the similarity of Tommy's and my profiles. For my father these similarities were surprising discoveries, but for me they were a long-awaited connection to a sibling. Mac's words increased my desire to meet my brother.

Ironically, when we walked into the restaurant in Caribou, we were seated right next to a man my father apparently knew. "Who are these people with you, Mac?" My father looked at me with a humble and apologetic look, uncertain what to do.

"Very special friends. Very special," was all he could say. I understood his predicament and silently forgave him one more time.

After lunch we took the kids for ice cream, and all of us posed for more pictures. Later we returned to the campground and talked until dark. We embraced and said our good-byes. I explained that we would stay at the campground for a few more days of vacation and left it up to him what to do. I had crawled enough. With a lump in my throat, I watched him leave, not sure when or if we would see each other again. I was too perplexed to cry. So many things about this meeting had felt right. But there was still a large element of hesitation on his part. He still seemed afraid to let his forty-five-year-old son, who now lived in Buffalo, or his lady friend of fourteen years, in on this secret from his past.

I walked down to the waterfront beyond our campsite and looked across the mirrorlike lake touched with a hint of orange from the setting sun. There I remained for a while trying to absorb all of the day's events. My daughter joined me, and I was soothed by the presence of her small frame nestled on my lap. The sun finally sank, giving way to the darkness and solace of a summer evening. We returned to our campsite where I began making preparations for the night.

It wasn't long before I caught sight of a beige car approaching. I watched intently; were my eyes deceiving me? He had returned! He jumped out of the car grinning, this time accompanied by his dog, Pepper. He opened the trunk and pulled out Annie's old plastic water dish. We had left it in his car at lunch. What a lame excuse! Later he admitted that he had turned his car around two other times, but had changed his mind.

Suddenly he pulled out a framed picture and silently handed it to me, studying my face for a reaction. It was a picture of himself and a younger man. "This is your brother." No longer was he referring to Tommy as his son. Now he was "your brother."

I held the picture for a long time, searching for a resemblance and feeling the completion of my journey. Already I felt connected to Mac, and to his son. Somehow, this time, I knew it would work out. The concept of becoming a sister had been such a fantasy all my life. After meeting my other siblings, I had still felt like an only child; this time I was about to have a brother.

I looked into my father's face and smiled. I had finished my search for my birth parents, but now I was beginning a whole new adventure, connecting the roots of my past with my present. I locked my arm in his, and we walked to the camp chairs and sat down.

"I am glad you came back," I said.

Contributors

Me-K Ando is a videomaker, installation artist and writer who explores and interrogates her adopted Korean identity including issues of cultural and geographical displacement. Her video *living in half tones* has been screened at the Asian American Film Festival in New York and Los Angeles and her short story *The Trip Inside* won a Short Fiction Award context. She is the recipient of a Jerome Regional Film/Video grant, a Jerome Installation Commission, a 1994 Loft McKnight Award in Creative Prose, and a 1994 Diverse Visions Regional Interdisciplinary Grant. Her articles, essays and short stories have appeared in *COLORS* magazine, *Transpacific Magazine*, *Asian Pages* and *godzilla*. She is currently program manager for the Asian American Renaissance in St. Paul, MN.

Judy Ashkenaz is the mother of two daughters. She works as an editor and book designer in Brattleboro, Vermont, where she and her husband have lived since 1976. Long active in local and state politics, she currently serves on the town school board and as a justice of the peace. She has been an election-night commentator on local radio and an occasional columnist on education and related topics for the Brattleboro *Reformer*. She is gathering material for a book on attachment issues in older adopted children.

Carol Austin, writing under a pseudonym, writes of a specific, painful frame in her parenting process. This in no way reflects her daily life now as she delights in her two beautiful children and terrific partner. Both she and her partner are active, out parents and, because of their home-state's political environment, cautiously protect their biracial family.

Ruth Myra Bayer writes and teaches in the Boston area. She is designing a curriculum to teach Israeli and Palestinian literature to high-school students. She especially enjoys reading on her front porch in the sun and digging in her new garden.

Jody Lannen Brady teaches at George Mason University, where she received her M.F.A. in Creative Writing. Her short fiction has been published in several journals; excerpts of her novel set in the Amazon have appeared in the *Union Street Review*, the *Black River Review* and the *Hispanic Culture Review*. Her non-fiction includes essays and newspaper feature writing. She lives in Annandale, Virginia, with her husband, Bill, and her children, Matt and Kelly.

Beth Brant is a Bay of Quinte Mohawk from Tyendinaga Mohawk Territory in Ontario. She is the editor of *A Gathering of Spirit: Writing and Art by*

North American Indian Woman (Firebrand Books, and Women's Press, Canada, 1984), and the author of *Mohawk Trail* (Firebrand Books and Women's Press, 1985) and *Food & Spirits* (Firebrand Books and Press Gang, Canada, 1991). Her work has appeared in numerous Native, feminist and lesbian anthologies and she has received an Ontario Arts Council award, a Canada Council grant and is a recipient of a National Endowment for the Arts Literature Fellowship. She is a mother and a grandmother and lives with her partner of eighteen years, Denise Dorsz. She has been writing since the age of forty and considers it a gift for her community.

Laura Cunningham is the author of two published novels, *Sweet Nothings* (Doubleday, 1977) and *Third Parties* (Coward McCann and Geoghegen, 1980), and a memoir, *Sleeping Arrangements* (Knopf and New American Library), that was excerpted in *The New Yorker*. As a journalist she has been published by *The New York Times*, *Esquire*, *Newsday*, *The Village Voice* and hundreds of other periodicals. Her fiction has appeared in *The New Yorker*, *The Atlantic Monthly*, *Vogue* and literary quarterlies. Her *New York Times* "Hers" columns have been widely reprinted and anthologized. She is also a playwright, an adoptive mother and lives in New York City.

Susan Misao Davie is a photographer living in Seattle (but hopes to move to the country soon) with her husband and two children. She is currently involved in a writers' group for adopted women, and in the creation of a democratic school in Seattle. She has searched for, found and contacted her birth mother and birth father and all five of her half-siblings. None of these contacts have led to any fruitful relationships.

Kathleen Scully Davis lives, works and writes in Oakdale, Minnesota, where she has been a single mom for over twenty years. She spends intensive energy in her day job as a vocational counselor helping single parents obtain training, employment and self-sufficiency. She is a member of the Midwest Fiction Writers, the Loft for Writers and the Romance Writers of America. She and her sister, Mary, have collaborated on and completed their first novel. She enjoys reading (omnivorously), writing, cross-stitching, tea with friends, and the "sleep that knits the ravelled sleeve of care."

Lorraine Dusky is the author of *Birthmark* (M. Evans, 1979), the first book about the trauma of surrendering a child for adoption. Published in 1979, its controversial message spearheaded the debate about closed birth records and their impact on all parties in the adoption triangle. She is an award-winning journalist, co-author of *The Best Companies for Women* (Simon and Schuster, 1988) and author of the soon-to-be-published *Still Unequal: Women and the Law*. She and her daughter, Jane, have been reunited since 1981 and enjoy a loving and close relationship.

Louise Erdrich, a member of the Turtle Mountain Band of Chippewa, was raised in Wahpeton, North Dakota, the eldest of seven children. She is the author of the best-selling, award-winning novels, *Love Medicine* (Bantam, 1987), *The Beet Queen* (Henry Holt and Co., 1986), *Tracks* (Henry Holt and Co., 1988), *The Bingo Palace* (HarperCollins Publishers, Inc., 1994) and co-author with her husband, Michael Dorris, of *The Crown of Columbus* (HarperCollins Publishers, Inc., 1992), a novel, and *Route Two* (Lord John, 1992), a collection of their travel essays. Her most recent non-fiction is *The Blue Jay's Dance, A Birth Year* (HarperCollins Publishers, Inc., 1995). Her fiction has been honored by the National Book Critic's Circle and *The Los Angeles Times* and has been translated into fourteen languages. Her short stories have been selected for O'Henry Awards and for inclusion in the annual *Best American Short Story* anthologies.

Florence Fisher is the author of the ground-breaking 1973 adoption memoir *The Search For Anna Fisher* (Arthur Fields Books, 1973). As president and founder of the Adoptees' Liberty Movement Association she is a national leader in the adoptee search and reform movement within the United States and abroad. She lives in New York City.

Robyn Flatley is a forty-seven-year-old political eco-feminist painter, videographer, filmmaker, poet and writer who is currently living in Brattleboro, Vermont.

Patricia Fox: As the sun rises over the tranquil mountains of western Maine, she wakes up, says goodbye to her husband, awakens her two children and begins her day. As she opens the door to the high school, she contemplates how she will bring up today's gender topics. Known as a rebel (with causes) she walks through the hall smiling and greeting students, pausing to tease or joke. Enthusiastically, she enters her classroom, spends the day instructing in the areas of English and theater, pausing occasionally to reflect on her own writing. At home, she sometimes is rewarded with a letter or phone call from her birth father or brother. As the sun sets, she gets in her vehicle, brainstorming for the evening's play rehearsal.

Marian Modelle Howard is a psychotherapist with practices in New York City and Saugerties, New York. She has written short stories and poetry and is currently working on a novel. A student of Gurdjieff's teaching for the past five years, she has recently become interested in Tibetan Buddhism.

Her relationship with her younger daughter continues to develop. She hopes one day to be in contact with her older daughter.

Kai Jackson is currently working on a Ph.D. in African-American Studies at Emory University, Atlanta, Georgia. She writes fiction and beads jewelry in her spare time.

Denise Sherer Jacobson is a California transplant from her 1950s birthplace of the Bronx, New York. Whether she writes of growing up in the '50s and '60s, being Jewish, having cerebral palsy, or exploring adulthood and motherhood, Sherer Jacobson attempts to clear away some of the prejudice, fear and ignorance which obstruct the path to compassion, strength and freedom. Her published works include "American Bandstand" (*Prejudice*, Hyperion Press, 1995), features in *The East Bay Express* and pieces in national literary magazines. She makes her home in the Bay Area with her husband Neil and eight-year-old David.

Jackie Kay was born in Edinburgh in 1961 and brought up in Scotland. She received an Honours Degree in English from the University of Stirling in 1983. Her first collection of poetry, *The Adoption Papers* (Bloodaxe, 1991) won an Eric Gregory award, a Scottish Arts Council Award, a Forward Poetry award and a Saltire award and has been broadcast on radio. Her second collection of poetry, *Other Lovers*, published by Bloodaxe in 1994 received the Somerset Maugham Award. She has also published two volumes of children's poetry, *Two's Company* and *Three Has Gone* (1995) and has written plays and works for television. She lives in London.

Wendy Lichtman is a freelance writer living in Berkeley, California, with her husband and two children. Her personal essays appear in local and national magazines, and she has written four books of fiction for young adults.

Nancy Mairs grew up in New England and holds an M.F.A. in creative writing (poetry) and a Ph.D. in English from the University of Arizona. She has taught writing at the University of Arizona and UCLA. Her recent books include three collections of essays: *Plaintext* (University of Arizona Press, 1992); *Carnal Acts* (HarperCollins, 1990); *Voice Lessons: On Becoming a (Woman) Writer* (Beacon Press, 1994); a memoir, *Remembering the Bone House: An Erotics of Place and Space* (Harper & Row, 1989); and a spiritual autobiography, *Ordinary Times: Cycles in Marriage, Faith, and Renewal* (Beacon Press, 1993). Her current project is titled, *Waist-High in the World: (Re)Constructing (Dis)Ability*. She and her husband, George, a high-school English teacher, live in Tucson.

Catherine E. McKinley is co-editor of *Afrekete: An Anthology of Black Lesbian Writing* (Anchor Books, 1995). She lives in Brooklyn, New York, and is currently working on a novel, *Chewing the Naval String*, about the coming of age of a transracial adopted woman.

Jacquelyn Mitchard is a writer, author and speaker who divides her time between freelance journalism, creative projects and work as a senior writer at the University of Wisconsin. She is a contributing editor to *Parenting* magazine, a correspondent for *Money Magazine* and writes regularly for other journals including *TV Guide, Glamour, Woman's Day*, and *Self*. A 1994 Ragdale Foundation Fellow and recipient of 1993 and 1994 Maggie Awards for excellence in public-service magazine journalism, she is the author of *Mother Less Child: The Love Story of a Family* (W.W. Norton, 1985) and *Jane Addams of Hull House* (Gareth Stevens Press). A novel, *The Deep End of the Ocean*, will be published by Viking Press in 1996. She lives in Madison, Wisconsin with her four children, ranging in age from five to nineteen. Her late husband was the award-winning Wisconsin journalist Dan Allegretti.

Merril Mushroom has been an adoptive/foster parent since 1969. She has five adopted children. She has written training materials for adoption/foster care workers and teaches children who have special needs. She lives and works in the rural South.

Priscilla T. Nagle lives with her husband in the outback of northeast Arizona, beyond power lines of any kind. She is the mother and stepmother of seven marvelous young people. Her oldest son has recently enriched her life by reuniting with her and his two brothers. Having spent years trying to be a scientist, she is now admitting she has always been a writer and musician, and is currently completing three of her stories.

Artemis OakGrove is the author of lesbian erotic novels, The Throne Trilogy, published by Lace Publications: *The Raging Peace* (1984), *Dreams of Vengeance* (1985) and *Throne of Council* (1986). She is also the author of *Nighthawk* (Lace Publications, 1987), *Led Astray* (Tickerwick, 1994), *Warclouds* (1995) and a forthcoming novel, *Secrets*. She is currently writing a book of original bead work projects, co-authoring a guide to lesbian erotica and developing a World Wide Web page for bead sources.

Minnie Bruce Pratt has published three books of poetry, *The Sound of One Fork* (Night Heron Press, 1981), *We Say We Love Each Other* (Firebrand Books, 1992) and *Crime Against Nature* (Firebrand Books, 1990), chosen by the Academy of American Poets for the 1989 Lamont Poetry selection (an annual award given for the best second full-length book of poetry by a U.S. author), the 1991 American Library Association Gay and Lesbian Book Award for Literature and nominated for a Pulitzer Prize in Poetry. In 1991 Pratt, along with lesbian writers Crystos and Audre Lorde, received the Lillian Hellman/Dashiell Hammett awards given by the Fund for Free Expression. She is also the author of *Rebellion: Essays 1980-1991* (Firebrand Books, 1991) and a book of prose stories, *S/HE* (Firebrand Books, 1995). Pratt lives in the New York City metropolitan area and is on the graduate faculty of The Union Institute, a non-residential alternative university.

Sheila Rule is a reporter for *The New York Times*. As a journalist she has been a foreign correspondent and has written about events in Africa and Europe. She currently writes about popular music and lives in New York City with her six-year-old-son, Sean.

Shay Youngblood is author of the plays, *Shakin' the Mess Outta Misery* (Dramatic Publishing Company, 1989), and *Talking Bones* (Dramatic Publishing Company, date not yet set) and the collection of short stories, *The Big Mama Stories* (Firebrand Books). She is a teacher of multi-genre creative writing workshops and is currently at work on a novel. Ms. Youngblood is a member of the Writers Guild of America and the Dramatists' & Authors' Guild.

Acknowledgments

"A Long Story" from *Mohawk Trial* by Beth Brant. Copyright © 1985 by Beth Brant. Reprinted by permission of Firebrand Books.

"Sleeping Arrangements" excerpted from *Sleeping Arrangements* by Laura Cunningham. Copyright © 1986 by Laura Cunningham. Reprinted by permission of Alfred A. Knopf Inc.

Louise Erdrich's Foreword excerpted from *The Broken Cord: A Family's Ongoing Struggle with Fetal Alcohol Syndrome* by Michael Dorris. Copyright © 1989 by Michael Dorris. Reprinted by permission of HarperCollins Publishers, Inc.

"Somebody's Child" excerpted from *The Search for Anna Fisher* by Florence Fisher. Copyright © 1973 by Florence Fisher. Reprinted by permission of the author.

"The Adoption Papers" by Jackie Kay is reprinted by permission of Bloodaxe Books, Ltd. from: *The Adoption Papers* by Jackie Kay (Bloodaxe Books, 1991).

"Ron Her Son" from *Plaintext* by Nancy Mairs. Copyright © 1986 by Nancy Mairs. Reprinted by permission of University of Arizona Press.

"Mother to Mother" by Jacquelyn Mitchard was originally published in *Parenting* magazine. Reprinted with permission of *Parenting* magazine.

"All the Women Caught in Flaring Light," from *Crime Against Nature* by Minne Bruce Pratt. Copyright © 1990. Reprinted by permission of Firebrand Books.

"Sheila and Sean," by Sheila Rule from *The Single Mother's Companion: Essays and Stories by Women*, edited by Marsha R. Leslie. Copyright © 1994 by Marsha R. Leslie. Reprinted by permission of Seal Press.

"Did My Mama Like to Dance" and "They Tell Me . . . Now I Know" from *The Big Mama Stories* by Shay Youngblood. Copyright © 1989 by Shay Youngblood. Reprinted by permission of Firebrand Books.

The Women's Press is Britain's leading women's publishing house. Established in 1978, we publish high-quality fiction and non-fiction from outstanding women writers worldwide. Our exciting and diverse list includes literary fiction, detective novels, biography and autobiography, health, women's studies, handbooks, literary criticism, psychology and self help, the arts, our popular Livewire Books series for young women and the bestselling annual *Women Artists Diary* featuring beautiful colour and black-and-white illustrations from the best in contemporary women's art.

If you would like more information about our books or about our mail order book club, please send an A5 sae for our latest catalogue and complete list to:

The Sales Department
The Women's Press Ltd
34 Great Sutton Street
London EC1V 0DX
Tel: 0171 251 3007
Fax: 0171 608 1938

Also of interest:

Marijke Woolsey and Susan King, editors
Dear Mother
An Anthology of Women Writing To or About Their Mothers

With Alice Walker, Maya Angelou, Marilyn French, Catherine Cookson, Virginia Woolf, Stephanie Dowrick, Mary Daly, Marge Piercy, George Sand, Sylvia Plath, May Sarton, Audre Lorde and many more.

Introduced by Judith Arcana, author of *Every Mother's Son* and *Our Mothers' Daughters*.

In this warm, inspiring and compelling collection of letters, journal extracts and essays, leading women writers bring honest and heartfelt new perspectives to bear on the strength and significance of mother-daughter ties. Together they explore the enormous diversities and depths that make up a daughter's relationship with her mother.

'Inspiring . . . a revealing, pleasurable read.' *Options*

'A penetrating examination of motherhood . . . Brilliantly revealing.' *Sunday Telegraph*

'Warm and inspiring . . . A fine anthology.'
Evening Express

'Autobiographical writing at its best.' *Pink Paper*

'Outstanding.' Shena Mackay, *Financial Times*

Autobiographical Writings/Women's Lives £6.99
ISBN 0 7043 4345 2

Judith Arcana
Our Mothers' Daughters

With an introduction by Phyllis Chesler

Now a major, bestselling classic, *Our Mothers' Daughters* is Judith Arcana's groundbreaking and definitive book on the relationship between mothers and daughters. How we are socialised into roles which can set us in opposition to each other; our mothers' involvement in our training to be women; childhood patterns; competition; the pain of separation; the role of fathers; the conflicts that can and often do arise; and how we can develop better relationships with our mothers.

'Irresistibly moving and fascinating . . . I would urge you to read it.' Penny Vincenzi, *Cosmopolitan*

'Beautifully written . . . a welcome addition for any woman's bookshelf. Whether you read it as a mother or a daughter or both it might help you understand life a little better than before.' *Woman's World*

'About woman's stormiest, most tumultuous love affair: the one all daughters have with their mothers . . . *it blew my mind* . . . Already this precious little book, much thumbed and pored over, has passed among my friends and acquaintances.' Val Hennessey, *Honey*

'Please mother, read this book. It will make everything – everything – clear.' Phyllis Chesler

Psychology/Women's Studies £7.99
ISBN 0 7043 3864 5

Judith Arcana
Every Mother's Son
The Role of Mothers in the Making of Men

**'The boys: how can they withstand the pressure? How
can they say no to the gift of power? How can they turn a
deaf ear, a blind eye, to television, to the toys – to the
girly magazines? And what about the responsibility for all
of that? Must mothers of sons run interference on the
whole damn culture for our sons?'**

How can a mother care lovingly for a small boy, yet avoid
reinforcing the examples he receives from all around him? How
can she challenge male stereotypes, and at the same time fit him
to survive in the world in which we live? Can our sons grow up
to be our friends? Judith Arcana, author of the much-loved
bestseller *Our Mothers' Daughters*, faced these questions with her
own son, and has drawn on the diary she kept then, as well as on
interviews with other women, to write this moving, honest and
thought-provoking book.

'Truly wonderful.' Phyllis Chesler

Parenting/Psychology £8.99
ISBN 0 7043 3916 1

Marianne Grabrucker

There's a Good Girl

Gender Stereotyping in the First Three Years of Life – a Diary

When Marianne Grabrucker gave birth to her first child, she was
determined not to bring her up as a conventional 'girl'. But life
quickly proved more complex than early resolutions allowed.
Over the next three years of motherhood, Grabrucker charted
her daughter's development and the many ways in which she was
taught gender stereotypes – both by the world at large and
through her mother's own, inadvertent, example. The result was
this compelling diary, an instantaneous and enduring international
bestseller. The new edition features an afterword by the author
and her now thirteen-year-old daughter in which they reflect on
the decisions made.

**'It is a ray of light in a fog – and deserves to be read by all
parents who feel foxed by their children's grim
determination to cling to gender roles from which their
parents think they have protected them.'
Polly Toynbee, *Guardian***

Parenting/Biography £6.99
ISBN 0 7043 4090 9

Joan Ryan
Little Girls in Pretty Boxes
The Making and Breaking of Elite Gymnasts and Figure Skaters

Gymnastics and figure skating are seen as the most magical and enchanting of international sports, captivating television audiences around the world. Their stars are lauded as storybook princesses, blessed with poise, beauty, agility and grace. But at what cost to the young women themselves?

In this superb, acclaimed book, award-winning sports journalist, Joan Ryan, reveals the enormous pressures to perform placed on young gymnasts and figure skaters today. Enduring punishing training schedules and often competing in the face of severe and debilitating injuries, these aspiring stars are also required to conform to outdated ideals of femininity, with pre-pubescent physiques essential to sporting success. As the race for Olympic gold becomes a race against womanhood, Ryan documents the commonality of eating disorders, restricted growth, weakened bones and damaged psyches among these elite athletes. *Little Girls in Pretty Boxes* reveals the frightening truth about how young women are routinely sacrificed on the road to gymnastic and ice-skating success.

'This book will change for ever the way we look at these most beloved of sports.' Billie Jean King

'A must read.' *Los Angeles Times*

Women's Studies/Sport £8.99
ISBN 0 7043 4488 2

The Women's Press Handbook Series

Gerrilyn Smith
The Protectors' Handbook
Reducing the Risk of Child Sexual Abuse and Helping Children
Recover

How much more effective would we be in working against child
sexual abuse if every adult had the knowledge currently available
only to professionals?

With child sexual abuse now unquestionably widespread, every
adult in contact with children must – and can – be an active
protector. Now, in this unique and essential book, child
psychologist Gerrilyn Smith gives adults all the information and
skills needed to protect children in their day-to-day lives.
Drawing on her many years of professional experience in the
field, a wide range of sources and proven techniques – as well as
the experiences of young survivors themselves – she offers a fully
comprehensive, practical and step-by-step guide to recognising,
reducing the risks of and overcoming the effects of abuse.

From being aware of the many possible signs of abuse to helping a
child confide, from creating the best context for recovery to
finding the most appropriate professional help, this urgently
needed, accessible book is absolutely essential reading for
every adult.

Health/Self Help £6.99
ISBN 0 7043 4417 3

Ellen Prescott
Mondays Are Yellow, Sundays Are Grey
A Mother's Fight to Save Her Children From the Nightmare of
Sexual Abuse

Ellen Prescott's four-year-old daughter, Carolina, has colours for
the days of the week. Sunday – the day she visits her father – is
grey. Monday – when she won't be left alone with him for
another whole week – is yellow. *Mondays Are Yellow, Sundays Are
Grey* is Ellen Prescott's painstaking, detailed and heartrending
account of her discovery of the sexual abuse of her children and
her struggle to save them. She describes the strange, disturbed
behaviour of her children; her inability to comprehend and accept
the truth; her fight for help from disbelieving doctors, therapists
and friends; how she deals with her damaged, distressed and
confused children; the impending court battle to keep her
husband away from them; and the healing and recovery that
eventually comes.

Including a highly positive and affirming afterword from Carolina,
the eldest daughter, *Mondays Are Yellow, Sundays Are Grey* is a
crucial and invaluable book in the process of understanding
mothers' and children's experience of abuse, and a book that
every parent, professional and woman should read.

Health/Women's Studies/Self-Help £8.99
ISBN 0 7043 4483 1

Louise Armstrong
Rocking the Cradle of Sexual Politics
What Happened When Women Said Incest

After years of secrecy and denial, how did incest become the
routine, banal subject it is today – the standard fare of talk shows
and celebrity interviews? How did we move from total
incredulity, to a brief moment of belief in the testimony of
women and children – back to a point where False Memory
Syndrome and reports of satanic abuse are only the latest in a
long line of contradictory media revelations? And what are the
implications of this for women and children?

Challenging the accepted wisdom that incest can be viewed
simply as a personal problem requiring 'treatment' and 'help',
Louise Armstrong – author of the groundbreaking *Kiss Daddy
Goodnight* – charts the emergence of an opportunistic growth
industry of self-proclaimed healers and professionals. She reveals
how the truth in what women and children are saying has been
distorted by a cacophony of 'expert' voices and media exposés.
Uncovering the many ways in which incest has been defused as an
issue, *Rocking the Cradle of Sexual Politics* provides a crucial and
much-needed new perspective on one of the most vital issues for
women today and argues the need for a renewed political
awareness and engagement as our only hope for lasting change.

Sexual Politics £8.99
ISBN 0 7043 4460 2

Lois Keith, editor
Mustn't Grumble
Writing by Disabled Women

Winner of the MIND Book of the Year Award

Controversial, humorous, hard-hitting and moving, *Mustn't Grumble*
is the most powerful and far-ranging book ever to be published on
disability and illness. From access to abuse, equality to equanimity,
this is an honest, eloquent and hilarious collection. Published as the
issue of disability at last began to reach prominence in social, political
and cultural debate, *Mustn't Grumble* won huge acclaim and became
one of the most talked about books of the decade. Now required
reading on courses and training programmes, *Mustn't Grumble* gives a
superb insight into the lives and the most pertinent issues for
disabled women and is essential reading for every disabled and non-
disabled individual.

'An alternately hilarious and powerful collection . . . Honest,
eloquent and humorous.' *Sainsbury's – The Magazine*

'Sometimes shocking and controversial, it's also very
honest and sometimes hilarious. Highly recommended.'
Living

'A powerful range of voices.' *Guardian*

'Inspiring reading. Besides fear, pain and anger, they reveal
joy, humour and a vibrant insistence for quality of life.'
Woman's Realm

'Brings into focus many powerful, sensitive and exceedingly
personal issues . . . This humorous, sometimes shocking,
but optimistic book goes straight to the heart.' *Herald*

Autobiography/Disability £7.99
ISBN 7043 4344 4